Neti:
Healing Secrets of
Yoga and Ayurveda

By David Frawley

LOTUS
PRESS

DISCLAIMER

This book is not intended to treat, diagnose or prescribe. The information contained herein is in no way to be considered as a substitute for a consultation with a duly licensed health care professional.

Cover image courtesy of Hinduism Today

Cover & Page Design/Layout: Susan Honeywell, LJ Graphics

Sivani Alderman - editing and proofing

First Edition, 2005

Printed in the United States of America

Neti: Healing Secrets of Yoga and Ayurveda includes bibliographical references.

ISBN: 978-0-9409-8585-8

Library of Congress Control Number: 2005922225

Published by:
Lotus Press, PO Box 325, Twin Lakes, WI 53181 USA
web: www.lotuspress.com
e-mail: lotuspress@lotuspress.com
800-824-6396

Table of Contents

Preface

Today, Yoga classes can be found in almost every community in America. They are part of a general search for better health, vitality and awareness that is rapidly becoming an important part of our culture. Along with this search for greater well-being is an exploration of various methods of detoxification and internal cleansing. We cannot expect to feel better as long as our body is clogged with the pollutants and pathogens that can cause disease. Internal cleansing is probably the first step towards a healthier life, which includes not only special detoxification measures of a clinical nature but daily hygienic practices that everyone can do.

In this regard, the Yoga tradition offers us another important tool of self-healing, a special device called a 'neti pot' and a process of cleansing the nostrils or 'nasal irrigation' that it is used for. The use of this device is not only common to Yoga practitioners but is extending to the entire natural health community along with the use of herbs, massage and other alternative therapies. However, so far there is no single book which explains this important health tool, how to use it on a daily basis and its greater applications for the treatment of disease.

This small book has arisen to fill that need. Its purpose is twofold. The first is to introduce the neti pot and its usage to everyone at the basic level of daily hygiene. This will provide anyone new to this ancient method of nasal irrigation a simple key to its operation on a regular basis.

The second is to introduce an advanced therapeutic usage of the neti pot, showing how to use it along with herbs and oils and in conjunction with other healing methods in order to treat specific constitutional (mind-body) types and particular disease conditions. This information will be particularly useful to health care practitioners, especially to Yoga teachers and Ayurvedic practitioners.

The general usage of the neti pot is described both relative to ordinary health considerations and with reference to the Yoga system from which it arose. The therapeutic usage of the neti pot, on the other hand, is described in terms of Ayurvedic medicine, the traditional natural healing system of India, or what could be called 'yogic medicine'. I have tried to introduce the basics of Yoga and Ayurveda so that even a beginner can understand their relevance in the use of the neti pot.

Ayurvedic doctors frequently recommend the neti pot as part of right life-style considerations both for the prevention of disease and for the attainment of optimal energy. Many people who have gone to Ayurvedic practitioners have come away with the recommendation to use the neti pot for this reason, or have even been sold one by their therapist.

This book on the neti pot can be supplemented by my other books on Ayurvedic medicine like Ayurvedic Healing and Yoga and Ayurveda that provide more detail on the Ayurvedic view of health and yoga, which can only be alluded to here. For those wanting more information on the herbs referred to in the book, please examine my co-authored book, The Yoga of Herbs that contains a list of relevant western and Ayurvedic herbs and their uses. Yogic studies of the breathing process and pranayama (yogic breathing practices) can also be of help. Please consult your Yoga teacher or Ayurvedic practitioner for more details.

May this book help you breathe your way to a better life!

Dr. David Frawley

Santa Fe, New Mexico

March 2004

Part I

The Neti Pot and How to Use It

1.
The Neti Pot and the Practice of Nasal Irrigation

Have you ever suffered from not being able to breathe fully through your nose and wished that there were a simple way to just pour water through your nostrils and quickly open them? Perhaps you have tried a saline solution in your nose for this purpose, using the little vials from the drugstore that are available for this purpose, but found that it was not strong enough to produce the desired effect.

You should realize that there is a time-tested way to effectively clear the sinuses. This occurs through the use of a small pot of water, called a *neti pot*. You need no longer be a victim of sinus congestion or any other impaired nasal functioning, nor do you have to rely on decongestant drugs, that often have many side affects, in order to deal with such problems.

The neti pot is a small water pot specifically devised for cleansing the nasal passages – for the purposes of what could be called 'nasal irrigation'. You simply fill the pot with warm water along with a little salt and insert the spout or nozzle of the neti pot into your nostrils. You can then pour as much water through your nostrils as you like or as you need.

The neti pot originates from the Yoga tradition of India and its millennia old health and awareness traditions. The term neti, which originally means 'to guide', refers to the water that guides or draws our energy through the nasal passages, opening them up along the way.[1] The neti pot has long been used as an aid for Yoga practices, particularly to facilitate deep breathing. The neti pot, however, is not simply an ancient health secret. It is recommended by many modern naturopaths and doctors today. It is a simple but time-tested tool of personal hygiene that everyone can use with benefit. It can now be found not only at Yoga centers but also at natural food stores and herb stores in many locales throughout the country.

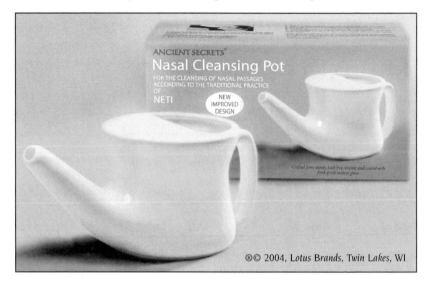

®© 2004, *Lotus Brands, Twin Lakes,* WI

The neti pot is usually ceramic, although traditional pots made of metal were also used. It looks like a small water pot for watering flowers and is usually less than a cup in size. It has a small spout that can be comfortably inserted into the nostrils in order to pour water through them.

The neti pot is a convenient device that one can take along even when traveling. Many people like to have one for travel and one to keep at home. One could say that it is as important for cleansing the nostrils as a toothbrush is for cleansing the teeth and should be a part of daily hygiene. After you use it regularly you will feel that your morning cleansing routine is incomplete without it.

The Poor Quality of Our Air

Even if you rarely suffer from overt sinus or nasal problems, the neti pot is still a great device for you to have. Our nasal passages filter the air that we breathe, which we take in during the course of the day in great volumes; however, it is rarely of the best quality for us to breathe!

The nose is perhaps our most-used organ in the body. It also has the most direct contact with our external environment and its many potential toxins and irritants. The nose has to filter dust, pollen and the many pollutants of our modern lives that we may not see or even always smell.

The nose has to deal with the outside air that may be too dry, too damp, too hot or too cold for the body. It has to adjust to our climate, which may be that of the seacoast, desert, mountains or other habitats that present their own special challenges. It must adapt to the many weather changes around us, including the effects of the wind that can be sudden and strong, particularly seasonal changes that may result in colds and flus.

The air of our urban environments brings in many of its own challenges. Our home and office environments also have heaters and air conditioners that we must deal with. There is probably no other organ in the body that has to adjust so quickly to such a range of different influences.

Just think of the chemicals, smog and smoke that many of us are exposed to on a regular basis in automobiles or outdoors in our cities. There are similar chemicals, artificial fragrances and recycled or stagnant air that we are exposed to in our offices, homes, in stores or in hotels. Most of the time, we are breathing air that is hardly ideal. Our nostrils are under extraordinary stress and an almost constant attack from many artificial substances that they were never evolved to deal with, as well as having to deal with the many natural forces that they were designed to handle.

Many of us suffer from respiratory ailments or reduced respiratory function because of the poor condition of our air, which can be the basis for many other health problems, from fatigue and depression to critical illnesses. Naturally, our sinuses are the first to get impacted by such air. Weakened sinuses often result in pain, particularly in the form of headaches, which can greatly reduce the quality and comfort of our lives. Sinus weakness or blockage can reduce our ability to work, to play or to make the best possible use of our energies in life, however we wish to use these. Unfortunately, although sinus problems are easy to note, they are also easy to overlook, neglect and do little or nothing about.

Mucus-forming Foods

Besides external sources of discomfort to the nose and sinuses there are equally important internal causes of sinus and lung problems. The main such internal cause is our modern diet, which contains large amounts of mucus-forming food. Mucus-forming foods include dairy products, breads, pastries, sweets, fats and fried foods of all types. Foods that are too greasy, sweet or salty will increase mucus.

Almost any junk food or fast food will tend to increase mucus in the body. Low carb diets help many people because they generally reduce the amount of mucus-forming foods that we consume. Overeating results in greater mucus production in the body, with the food that the stomach cannot digest easily turning into mucus. Bad food combinations such as too many sweets in conjunction with a protein meal generally cause mucus as well.

Many of the beverages we drink increase mucus in the body. The worst in this regard are soft drinks. Milk can also do this as well as fruit juices taken with the meals. Additionally, any excess use of cold or ice water also has this effect.

One of the primary places that excess mucus will accumulate is in the head, which naturally produces a lot of mucus to protect the nasal and sinus passages and filter the air that we breathe. Excess mucus in the head can block the sinuses and impair our breathing process just as effectively as any external pollutants. *If we add the combined effects of both a mucus-forming diet and an exposure to bad or polluted air, this mucus problem in the head will be multiplied.*

The sedentary life-styles that most of us lead contribute to the build-up of mucus in the body from dietary and environmental factors. Poor circulation due to lack of exercise prevents the proper discharge of mucus. Too much time spent sitting or lying down contributes to this condition of stagnation in the body and the mind that allows such toxins to build up.

At the same time, many of us work with computers and information technology that requires us to have a clear head in order to do our work well. Our energy is focused in our head and eyes throughout the workday, which in turn puts more pressure on the sinuses. It is easy to see that our current cultural prescription of polluted air, poor diet, lack of exercise and excessive mental work puts our health at risk starting with the nose itself.

In addition to this, many of us may have deviated septums, neck problems, allergies or other health complications that can negatively impact our nostrils and their ability to do their work even under optimal circumstances.

The Role of the Neti Pot in Protecting the Nostrils

While we change or clean the filters on our vacuum cleaners or other machines and motors regularly; we neglect the most important filter in the body, which are the sinuses. The use of the neti pot enables us to cleanse this filter of the nasal passages so that they can work better and more efficiently. It helps remove any mucus from the body that we are producing through wrong diet or poor life-style, and which is lodged in the head.

The neti pot is an important and powerful tool for cleaning the sinuses, which is relevant for anyone seeking to improve their health, sharpen their mental and sensory acuity, increase their breathing capacity or strengthen their general vitality in any manner. It is a wonderful means to raise the levels of both physical and mental energy – to promote the flow of positive vitality through the mind, senses and heart and through the entire respiratory, circulatory and nervous systems.

Everyone can benefit from the daily usage of the neti pot, particularly first thing in the morning. It is often better than a cup of coffee or hot tea for waking us up, for stimulating the mind and for helping us get going on our daily routine. After trying it and using it for a few days, you are likely to continue with it as a life-long practice and wonder how you got along without it.

If you feel sluggish in the morning, if you have any difficulty breathing, if your tongue has any significant coating – these are all signs that you can benefit from nasal irrigation for cleansing and clearing the passages of the head.

Detoxification, Weight Reduction and Rejuvenation

The neti pot is commonly used by yoga students and practitioners on a daily basis as part of a yogic way of life. Anyone who wishes to benefit from yoga postures, breathing practices or meditation will want to try it out, as will be explained in more detail later in the book. But its value goes far beyond yoga.

There are very few of us who do not suffer from some daily or seasonal sinus congestion, dryness, or headaches, which can all be effectively treated through use of the neti pot. It is also very helpful for dealing with colds, flu, asthma and related pulmonary diseases, though it requires greater caution and expertise in its usage for these more acute conditions.

The neti pot aids in expelling excess mucus from the entire body, starting with the nostrils and sinuses, which often serve as a lid to hold mucus in the body. It sets in motion an entire bodily process for removing mucus by opening up the circulation of air and energy throughout the circulatory and nervous systems, which in turn will affect digestion and all other bodily systems. For anyone suffering from excess mucus or lymphatic congestion, the neti pot is an important aid to better health.

Owing to its mucus-reducing and circulation-promoting actions, the neti pot can be an important part of any detoxification therapy. It can be as important as, and is easier to do than, colonics, liver flushes, and the many other detoxification measures that are popular today. It can also be done along with such detox therapies in order to improve their effects. We should not forget cleansing the sinuses in the head while we take care of cleansing the other organs and systems in the body such as our digestive tract.

As a means of improving our energy and circulation, the use of the neti pot can even be an important tool for weight loss. If our sinuses are blocked or impaired, our entire energy, circulation and digestion can become sluggish. This can result in the accumulation of excess weight or toxins in the body. For any weight reduction approach, the neti pot is an important aid to consider since it is a good adjunct to weight-reducing diets of various types.

In terms of improving our energy, the neti pot is good for those who want to increase their overall mental or physical functioning. Improving the power of the breath, it is good for athletes and for helping with outdoor activities. If we end up breathing through the mouth when we exert ourselves physically, this is a sign that our nostrils need such cleansing and strengthening. Clearing the senses, the neti pot is good for any mental, artistic or creative work. It brings fresh air and space to the brain and mind, providing a new energy for them to work.

As a means of improving our energy and our breathing capacity, the neti pot is also an important tool for helping us live longer. It is a powerful aid for any rejuvenation therapies that require renewed vital energy. We should not overlook its importance in helping us counter the aging process and promote longevity since it opens us up to more of the healing energy of life.

In clearing the head and sinuses, the use of the neti pot can help us deal with even the psychological blockages that reduce the quality of our lives. Emotional disturbances of anger, fear, anxiety, irritability or depression are often linked to poor breathing patterns and reduced functioning of the nostrils. Clearing the nostrils with the neti pot can add to our psychological well-being and give us some breathing space to deal with our emotional issues in life!

One of the problems in health care today is that we tend to rely too much on prescription drugs or clinical therapies rather than doing what we ourselves can do in our daily lives to improve our own health. The neti pot is one such tool that can help us be more independent and in control of our own health care. While it is no substitute for a doctor or for necessary medication, it can help us avoid unnecessary drugs and therapies. The neti pot is certainly worth the small effort required to use it and unlike drugs and more complex medical procedures it is safe, easy to do and without any significant side-effects.

Can You Benefit from Using a Neti Pot?

This question can be best answered by a simple experiment. Try breathing deeply, first with both nostrils together, then with each nostril separately (close the opposite nostril with a little finger pressure in order to do this). If you feel any blockage or reduction in the air flow, you can benefit from nasal cleansing through the use of a neti pot.

Check your nostrils not just during the day, when they are more likely to be fully open, but also as soon as you get up in the morning and just before you go to sleep at night, which are the two main times during the day that blockages are evident. But if you have problems with them at any time of the day, the neti pot can help you. There will be very few people for whom this is not the case!

Individuals who have to blow their nose frequently during the day will find that the neti pot can significantly reduce their need to do so. Those individuals who often have mucus draining down during the day, particularly dripping from the sinuses into the throat, will note that problem is reduced as well. Many will find that the use of the neti pot helps them breathe again, as if for the first time, allowing them to feel revitalized and renewed.

How important is such daily cleansing of the nostrils as compared with brushing or flossing of the teeth? Probably more significant because it improves our overall energy, while flossing the teeth is of more hygienic value, which cleansing the nostrils also has. Remember that we breathe through our nose all the time, while we only eat occasionally.

The neti pot is certainly worth a try in these days of rapidly rising health care costs. It is one of the least expensive and most effective forms of self-treatment relative to the time and effort that it requires!

2.
An Introduction to Yoga

To understand the value of using a neti pot, let us first examine the ancient healing systems in which its usage first arose. The neti pot dates back hundreds, if not thousands of years in the history of India. Both the Yoga tradition and its related Ayurvedic healing approach possess a broad array of internal cleansing techniques for both body and mind. The neti pot is part of their overall emphasis on helping us purify ourselves in order to arrive at physical, mental and spiritual well-being in life.

Yoga originally arose as a complete system of human development, showing us how to balance and harmonize body, breath, speech and mind in order to not only reach our full individual potential, but also to take us beyond the body to a greater oneness with the entire universe. As such, the practice of Yoga begins with the body as the first step in an extended process of internal growth, which helps us discover our true Self that is cosmic in nature.

The Greater System of Yoga

To this end, classical Yoga devised a comprehensive system of internal transformation in eight steps, taking us from the physical body to the highest consciousness.[2] These consist of:

1. Right life-style values (yama)
2. Right life-style observances (niyama)
3. Yoga postures (asana)
4. Yogic breathing (pranayama)
5. Control of the senses (pratyahara)

6. Concentration (dharana)
7. Meditation (dhyana)
8. Absorption (samadhi)

These eight aspects of Yoga begin with two related principles of right life-style values and right life-style observances (yama and niyama in Sanskrit). These consist of physical and mental purity, ethical living and a responsible interaction with both our human and natural environments. The yogic principles of right living include proper diet and purity of body, speech and mind. They provide the foundation for an awareness-promoting lifestyle that helps reduce suffering for all creatures.

The yamas or right life-style values consist of non-violence, truthfulness, responsible use of sexual energy, non-stealing and non-hoarding. The niyamas or right life-style observances consist of self-discipline, self-study, devotion to God, purity (including pure diet) and contentment. Yogic and Ayurvedic practices to cleanse and detoxify the body come in at this level, including the use of the neti pot and the general recommendation of a vegetarian diet.[3]

On the basis of a yogic life-style, Yoga developed a system of exercises or yoga postures (asanas) for harmonizing the physical body as its third step. Yoga postures aim at releasing stress and removing toxins from the joints, muscles and bones, at strengthening our digestive and circulatory capacities and increasing our overall adaptability and flexibility. To this end dozens of Yoga postures are taught in classes and adapted on an individual basis. For many people, Yoga asanas are their gateway to the world of Yoga and provide the foundation for physical health and ease of movement. Yoga asanas help cleanse all the organs and systems of the body and can be used along with various methods of physical detoxification.

This yogic harmonization of the body in turn is the basis for expanding the energy of the breath and the vital force within us through yogic breathing practices called pranayama, which is the fourth step or phase of Yoga practice. Pranayama not only gives us a better lung capacity and strengthens the heart; it also helps us to release disturbed emotions, agitating impressions and negative thoughts from the mind. Through it we can link our own life-energy with the universal life force and its healing powers on all levels. The neti pot is a key tool for preparing the body for the practice of pranayama, as we will discuss later in the sixth chapter of the book.

The yogic harmonization of the vital force provides the basis for harmonizing and controlling our senses through yogic sensory exercises and disciplines called pratyahara, the fifth aspect of eightfold Yoga. Pratyahara consists of relaxing the motor organs, refraining from unnecessary expression, avoiding excessive stimulation to the senses and replacing our agitated mental field of impressions with a pattern of harmony and compassion. It is particularly important for healing the mind, particularly in the modern world in which we suffer from stress and sensory overload.

This yogic harmonization of the senses enables us to control and develop our minds through a threefold practice of concentration (dharana), meditation (dhyana) and absorption (samadhi), the last three and most important of the eight limbs of Yoga.

Yogic concentration methods (dharana), like focusing on a mantra or geometrical design (yantra), help us develop our power of attention and one-pointedness of mind so that we can use our mental instrument, our mental muscle as it were, with as much skill as any other muscle of the body. Through yogic concentration we can give our full attention to whatever issue in life we need to deal with, which creates the internal space for solutions to our problems to come from within.

Yogic meditation exercises (dhyana), focusing on God or the higher Self, direct this concentrated awareness internally to change the very nature of our consciousness from limited to unlimited. They help us release deep-seated traumas, negative karmic patterns and egoistic fixations from our subconscious mind so that we can function in the world with full awareness, considerate of all beings.

Yoga leads us finally to a state of absorption or oneness (samadhi) in which we can empathize with, understand and find the truth of whatever we come into contact with, starting with our own deeper Self and Being. Through this yogic state of oneness we can experience all people and all of nature as different facets of our own deeper reality. Such a state of unity is the most powerful factor of both self-healing and self-transformation.

While modern Yoga usually emphasizes the asana or posture component of the system, one should remember that this is just one step or phase of a longer movement. It is but one rung of a greater ascent into consciousness, a creation of well-being on all levels of our existence in this magical universe of matter, energy, information and consciousness!

Traditional yoga generally regards Prana, breath or vital energy as its primary component, which is dealt with in great detail in various yogic texts.[4] This is because Prana is the prime force for healing the body, for controlling the senses and for concentrating the mind. It is the very power, or Shakti, of Yoga.[5] Pranayama is the most central aspect of Yoga and mediates between outer physical and life-style factors and inner meditation practices, providing us the energy necessary for both.

This yogic science of Prana is particularly stressed in *Hatha Yoga*, which is the main yogic approach for dealing with the physical body, while the yogic science of meditation is more the basis of *Raja Yoga* or higher yoga practices. We will examine the concept of Prana and Pranic healing in detail in the next chapter of this book.

The Neti Pot and Hatha Yoga

The neti pot derives from the tradition of Hatha Yoga, which first outlined its usage in detail.[6] Great Hatha Yoga gurus from ancient figures like legendary Yogi Gorakhnath to modern teachers like Swami Vishnudevananda have taught their students how to use the neti pot as an integral part of their daily discipline.

The term 'Hatha' itself arises from 'ha' referring to the sun and 'tha' meaning the moon. It indicates balancing the solar and lunar or masculine and feminine energies of the body and mind. This occurs through balancing the flow of the breath through the right and left nostrils, which are connected to the solar and lunar currents in the body, the *Pingala* and *Ida Nadis* of yogic thought that we will discuss later in the book. In this regard, the usage of the neti pot is a key tool for balancing the male and female energies within us, including balancing the right and left hemispheres of the brain.

Traditional Hatha Yoga simplifies the eight limbs of Yoga to three primary factors of asana (yoga postures), pranayama (yogic breathing exercises) and meditation, including the arousal of the Kundalini or inner power of Yoga. While modern Hatha Yoga emphasizes its asana component, the other two aspects of Hatha Yoga are equally important. The neti pot can help us with all three, improving our posture and awareness through improving our vital energy.

3.
An Introduction to Ayurveda

Ayurveda is the sister science of Yoga, healing both body and mind. Traditional Yoga employs an Ayurvedic language and approach for diagnosing and treating both physical and mental diseases. It follows an Ayurvedic view for understanding the workings of both our physiology and psychology. Similarly, Ayurveda takes a yogic approach to heal the body and mind, relying on the same philosophy of working with nature and the methodology of promoting balance inwardly and outwardly. Ayurveda also uses yogic methods like pranayama and meditation for rejuvenation of body and mind. So we should always think of the two systems together, particularly for healing purposes. [7]

The Three Doshas

Ayurveda is based upon a theory of three primary forces, called *doshas* in Sanskrit, behind both health and disease – a concept similar to the biological humors of old Greek medicine. The simplest way to understand the doshas is that each consists of two of the five elements or primary states of matter. They are an extension of the five element theory.

Vata, which literally means wind, consists of air and ether elements. Pitta, which means that which cooks things, consists of fire and water elements. Kapha, which means that which holds things together, consists of water and earth elements.

1. VATA DOSHA is the air or life-force that moves through and is contained in the channels, joints and cavities of the body.

2. PITTA DOSHA is the fire or heat capacity that is held in the blood, bile, enzymes and oily liquids of the body.

3. KAPHA DOSHA is the water or vital fluids held in the linings of the skin, mucus membranes, organs and muscles that constitute the earth element in the body.

Yet apart from their role as the main forces behind the body, the three doshas serve to mark *the constitution or mind-body type of a person.* Generally, one of the three is predominate in the nature of a person, resulting in what are called *Vata* types, *Pitta* types or *Kapha* types in Ayurvedic medicine. For purposes of simplicity, these are also called "air types", "fire types" and "water types", according to their dominant element.

1. VATA TYPES are generally taller or shorter than average in height and thin in build and in bodily frame. They have weak or variable digestions and suffer physically most from cold, wind and dryness.

   Vatas are nervous, creative and expressive in temperament and suffer psychologically most from fear and anxiety. Their main strengths are their quick energy, their adaptability and willingness to change and grow.

2. PITTA TYPES are generally average in size and weight and wiry or muscular in build. They possess a strong appetite and good digestion, and suffer physically most from heat, dampness and sun.

   Pittas are assertive, aggressive or determined in temperament and suffer psychologically most from anger. Their main strengths are their internal heat and light, their insight and willingness to examine things thoroughly before committing to a plan of action.

3. KAPHA TYPES are generally shorter in height, but occasionally can be tall, have large frames and hold weight easily. They have steady appetites but usually slow metabolisms and suffer physically most from cold, dampness and lack of movement.

Kaphas are receptive, feeling oriented and steadfast in their temperaments and suffer psychologically most from attachment. Their main strengths are their good physical energy reserve, their emotional resilience and their patience.

Ayurvedic books contain various questionnaires, lists or constitutional tests so that you can determine your own type.[8] Or you can consult your local Ayurvedic practitioner who will do this for you. You may also reference the following Ayurvedic Constitution Chart:

Ayurvedic Constitution Chart

	VATA (AIR)	PITTA (FIRE)	KAPHA (WATER)
HEIGHT:	tall or very short	medium	usually short but can be tall and large
FRAME:	thin, bony	moderate, good muscles	large, well-developed
WEIGHT:	low, hard to hold weight	moderate	heavy, hard to lose weight
SKIN LUSTER:	dull or dusky	ruddy, lustrous	white or pale
SKIN TEXTURE:	dry, rough, thin	warm, oily	cold, damp, thick
EYES:	small, nervous	piercing, easily inflamed	large, white
HAIR:	dry, thin	thin, oily	thick, oily, wavy, lustrous
TEETH:	crooked, poorly formed	moderate, bleeding gums	large, well formed
NAILS:	rough, brittle	soft, pink	soft, white
JOINTS:	stiff, crack easily	loose	firm, large
CIRCULATION:	poor, variable	good	moderate

(continued on next page)

Ayurvedic Constitution Chart (continued)

	VATA (AIR)	PITTA (FIRE)	KAPHA (WATER)
APPETITE:	variable, nervous	high, excessive	moderate but constant
THIRST:	low, scanty	high	moderate
SWEATING:	scanty	profuse but not enduring	low to start but profuse
STOOL:	hard or dry	soft, loose	normal
URINATION:	scanty	profuse, yellow	moderate, clear
SENSITIVITIES:	cold, dryness, wind	heat, sunlight, fire	cold, damp
IMMUNE FUNCTION:	low, variable	moderate, sensitive to heat	high
DISEASE TENDENCY:	pain, debility	fever, inflammation	congestion, edema
DISEASE TYPE:	nervous	blood, liver	mucus, lungs
ACTIVITY:	high, restless	moderate	low, moves slowly
ENDURANCE:	poor, easily exhausted	moderate but focused	high
SLEEP:	poor, disturbed	variable	excess
DREAMS:	frequent, disturbed	moderate, colorful	infrequent, romantic
MEMORY:	quick but absent-minded	sharp, clear	slow but steady
SPEECH:	fast, frequent	sharp, cutting	slow, melodious

(*continued on next page*)

Ayurvedic Constitution Chart (continued)			
	VATA (AIR)	**PITTA** (FIRE)	**KAPHA** (WATER)
TEMPERAMENT:	nervous, changeable	motivated	content, conservative
POSITIVE EMOTIONS:	adaptability	courage	love
NEGATIVE EMOTIONS:	fear	anger	attachment
FAITH:	variable, erratic	strong, determined	steady, slow to change
TOTAL	**Vata**_____	**Pitta**_____	**Kapha**_____

Cleansing the Channels of the Head

Both Yoga and Ayurveda emphasize cleansing and protecting the openings or orifices in the head; the mouth, eyes, ears and nostrils. These are our main locations for taking in substances from the environment, whether food, air or sensory impressions. Since they are such important points of intake, we must carefully consider their condition as well as what is brought in through them. Of these openings, the nostrils are the most important, covering both the sense of smell and our intake of oxygen and prana that is our primary fuel source, which is why the neti pot is so important.

Ayurvedic medicine expands the yogic usage of the neti pot and turns it into a therapeutic tool, particularly for treating diseases of the head, nose, ears and throat. The neti pot is an important medical device in Ayurveda as well as a tool of personal hygiene. It is part of many Ayurvedic health practices and therapies that we will examine in the second section of the book.

4.
Prana and Pranic Healing

All life is a manifestation of the life-force, which is called *Prana* in Sanskrit, Chi or Qi in oriental medicine and many other names in various healing traditions. This life force is not simply a chemical construction, nor is it instinctual or blind in its action. Prana, according to the great yogis, is the profound natural intelligence that creates the entire universe and its many worlds and creatures. It carries all the wisdom of evolution for both body and mind. [9]

Prana creates the body in all its intricacy from a cellular level, guiding all growth processes. It is the basis of all healing and has a capacity for rejuvenation as well. In this chapter we will examine how the use of the neti pot relates to Prana and how it can be an important means of increasing Prana or promoting Pranic healing.

The term Prana itself comes from the Sanskrit root 'an' which means 'to breathe', from which the related Greek term 'animus' or 'soul' arises. To this root is added the prefix 'pra' meaning 'prior' or 'forward.' Prana is the basic propulsive force that drives all activities in the universe and which is rooted in consciousness. It is ultimately the breath of God.

Our individual Prana makes up the energy field that creates, sustains and operates the physical body. This pranic field extends to an area about twelve inches from the body [10] and forms our aura. This Pranic field is responsible for our digestive power, luster of the skin, acuity of the senses, dexterity of our motor organs, strength of the immune system and overall equilibrium of the physical organism. Maintaining its proper flow both within and around the body is a key to health and well-being on all levels.

Prana and Health

Prana as the energy of life is the primary force of healing. All healing methods involve bringing more Prana or healing energy into the body through different vehicles or modalities. The food that we eat carries a physically concentrated Prana, which is extracted during the process of digestion. Herbs stimulate or strengthen Prana to carry out different functional activities like sweating, circulation, urination and elimination and their healing effects. Bodywork brings in Prana through therapeutic touch that conveys the healing force (Prana) of the practitioner to the patient. Even counseling involves putting the client in contact with the healing awareness, knowledge and emotional strength, the life-wisdom of the counselor.

There are many avenues through which Prana comes into the body during the course of our ordinary activities. The most obvious is through the lungs during the process of respiration. Eating food is another way to bring in a heavier form of Prana. The skin also takes in Prana and has its own process of respiration. The senses all bring in some form of Prana and stimulate our vital energy in various ways. The mind brings in Prana or life energy as emotion and thought.

Similarly, our different forms of elimination serve to remove toxins or waste-materials not only from the body but also from Prana. Whether it is the discharge of mucus from the nose, exhaled breath from the lungs, sweat from the skin, or urine and feces, Prana is also cleansed and renewed through this process. To adequately consider all our intakes and outputs, as it were, we must consider the role of Prana, which is the main force behind bringing about all actions.

The Role of the Nostrils and Sinuses

The nasal passages are our doorways to life, our initial point of contact with the external air. They constitute the first phase of the breathing process on which our overall vitality depends. They are also one of our main points of vulnerability, where we contact the outside forces of the air, weather and environment that can bring in disease. Our life begins and ends with the breath, which first enters through the nostrils.

The sinuses work to filter the air so that the lungs can better absorb oxygen. They purify the air for the continued extraction of prana that occurs later in the lungs and heart. However, according to Ayurvedic medicine, the nostrils and sinuses have an additional function beyond this outer action. They are also the first place in the body at which Prana or energy is absorbed from the breath – and the most immediate.

Through the sinuses we absorb a subtle Prana or vital force that goes directly into the brain and senses, which serves to invigorate them – to, as it were, light up the light bulb of the brain and mind. This subtle Prana is not simply oxygen but an energy of life and awareness from the greater conscious universe. It connects us with the greater cosmic intelligence and vitality.

This means that if the sinuses are not functioning properly, our entire absorption of Prana will be inhibited from the first to the last stage. We will experience a 'pranic or energy block' from the initial moment of pranic entrance into the body. This will set in motion a negative process, a kind of entropy by which the other phases of pranic absorption will get impaired, resulting in lower energy, reduced vitality and poor functioning of different types. It can set the entire disease process in motion that can reach to the very root of our vital force. So it is very important that we keep the Prana flowing smoothly from the beginning, that we keep our nostrils at their optimal level of functioning.

If our sinuses are blocked and we are breathing from our mouths we will not get this subtle Prana which stimulates the mind. That is why if we are breathing through our mouths, we are more likely to feel dull or tired. Mouth breathing also more likely results in an increase of mucus in the body. Without air flow to clean them out, mucus will accumulate in the sinuses and nostrils as well.

The Prana in the Head

We can call this Prana absorbed in the sinuses the 'Prana in the head'.[11] The sinuses are connected to all five of the senses. The sinuses behind the eyes facilitate our visual process and help bring Prana to the eyes. The sinuses near the ears and the related Eustachian tubes support our auditory process, bringing Prana to the ears. The nostrils themselves directly affect the nose and our sense of smell, which itself is an important indicator of how well we are breathing. The nearby oral cavity governs our sense of taste through the tongue. And our entire sense of touch has many sensitive nerves in the face that are directly impacted by the Prana in the head, affecting our sense of touch throughout the body.

This means that if we are not properly absorbing Prana in the sinuses then all five of our senses will have a diminished function and become susceptible to disturbance and disease. As the senses are the basis of our overall input of information on which we depend for our actions, this will impact all that we do, think and say. It can cause us to choose the wrong food to eat, to not do the proper exercise, or even to make wrong choices about our lives that depend upon the proper functioning of the senses.[12]

Of course, the nose is the first sense organ to be affected by blockage of the sinuses. But the eyes are not far behind. When the sinuses are blocked as in the case of colds, flu's or allergies we quickly get swollen or watery eyes or headaches in the sinuses behind the eyes that affect our sense of sight and cause light sensitivity. Ear infections are a more long term problem but a particularly harmful result of sinus infections that can directly affect the brain.

Sinus problems are not limited to the sense organs but extend to the motor organs, particularly the vocal organs, whose proper function depends upon the right flow of air through the throat, nostrils and sinuses. Blocked sinuses and sore throats commonly go together. When we cannot speak properly, all our other expressions and actions suffer.

This Prana in the head affects the brain and the mind itself. When the sinuses are blocked we cannot receive our proper prana or even blood flow to the head and brain. This results in dullness of mind, sleepiness, mental disorientation and other forms of low mental energy. It also creates a low emotional energy that can result in depression, anxiety and other psychological problems, reducing our resilience in dealing with the many emotional challenges of life.

Many people who think they may have emotional and psychological problems may only have a problem of impaired breathing or sinus congestion. Alternatively, many of those who may have such problems will have them complicated by sinus congestion that can make any treatment more difficult. We should not overlook the role of Prana in treating either the body or the mind, starting with this Prana in the head. For this, the neti pot is the best device to help us get started.

The Sinuses and the Immune System

As the first place our body connects to the external air, the nostrils form the first bulwark of our immune systems. That is why colds and flu and the first stage of most febrile diseases usually begin in the head, commonly with a head cold. Weak or blocked sinuses make us susceptible to contagious diseases from the common cold to more serious fevers and infections.

If we want to protect our immune systems, proper care of the nostrils and sinuses is essential and is probably the first step that we need to take. This is particularly important in this modern age when we overuse antibiotics and many of us have weakened immune systems because of this. The neti pot is a good tool to help us improve our Prana and strengthen our immunity. Its regular usage will make us less likely to require antibiotics. Unlike antibiotics it will strengthen, rather than weaken, our natural immunity.

Pranic and Energy Healing

True healing is not just a matter of making physical or chemical adjustments to the body at an outer level. It requires a shift in our internal energy, bringing a more positive energy of life and healing, or more Prana. Pranic or energy healing is as important as any physical healing. Most Ayurvedic and Yogic healing is based upon this principle.

The neti pot is an important tool of Pranic and energy practices. It can be used along with other forms of energy work including massage, polarity therapy, cranio-sacral work and related methods, as well as all Ayurvedic and Yogic methods. It provides a good means not only of cleansing the nostrils, but also of cleansing Prana. Nasal irrigation provides a kind of 'pranic bath' for our vital force, which can be as refreshing and invigorating as our baths or showers for the body as a whole.

5.
How to Use the Neti Pot

The neti pot is simple and easy to use. It just takes a few trial runs to get used to it. As most of us have not poured water through our nostrils before, it will be a new experience and may require a little practice. Some may find it initially to be difficult. However, if you have a little patience, soon you will be able to use the neti pot almost as easily as you tie your shoes. Any initial discomfort will soon be overcome by the soothing sensation of your nostrils being cleansed and refreshed and your mind feeling clear and energized.

It is best to use the neti pot for at least one week on a trial basis, every morning, before deciding whether to do it regularly. If you have a history of severe sinus blockage, it may be more difficult for you to perform this method of nasal irrigation, as more water may be required to effectively open the nostrils at first. Nonetheless, once you have succeeded in getting the water to flow easily through your nose and felt the relief that this brings, you will be more than willing to make the small effort required to get the neti pot to work for you.

This process of nasal irrigation generally takes only about five minutes once you have learned how to do it. It does not require a lot of your time, particularly when compared to the many benefits that it brings.

Size and Shape of the Neti Pot

Neti pots come in different sizes and shapes and are made of different materials. In India neti pots made of steel or copper are common. They are usually large in size, with a capacity of up to two cups when full. They can provide enough water to irrigate both nostrils, with a long narrow spout to pour the water.

In America today, most neti pots are ceramic and smaller in size with a capacity of one cup or less, which is enough to sufficiently irrigate one nostril at a time. Some ceramic neti pots are short and flat, resembling the shape of an "Aladdin's lamp", which gives them less capacity to hold water. They have a long spout to make for easy use and comfortable insertion into the nose. Another major version looks more like a "teapot" with a spout. It has a slightly larger water-holding capacity, less tendency to spill and is easier to clean than the flatter-style pots. Both styles are widely available.[13] Make sure you choose a neti pot that has a size and shape that works well for you.

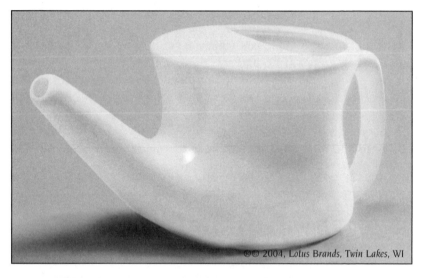

©© 2004, *Lotus Brands*, Twin Lakes, WI

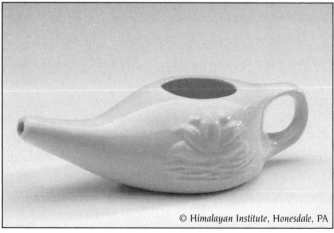

© *Himalayan Institute*, Honesdale, PA

How to Use the Neti Pot

Following I explain in detail how to use the neti pot, beginning with the preparation of the water solution to complications that may arise afterwards. Please study this material carefully if you are going to begin using the neti pot, as it should cover all the main considerations that may arise for you. If you are already using the neti pot regularly, this material is still important and may help you use it more efficiently.

The Water for the Neti Pot

The solution for the neti pot ordinarily consists of warm water with a little salt dissolved in it.

Warm water is soothing to the mucus membranes, which reflect body temperature and therefore works the best. Although the water used in the neti pot should be warm in temperature, it should not be so hot as to cause irritation.

You can test the water temperature with your finger first. The nostrils will be more sensitive to heat than the fingers, so if the water is hot to the touch, it will definitely feel uncomfortable when poured through the nose.

The chlorine used in tap water can be irritating for many people. Consequently many people prefer to use filtered, bottled or distilled water for the neti pot. This is particularly true for regular or long term use, which means the water will need to be heated first. Some people simply use warm tap water for this purpose.

However, cool water can at times be used for the neti pot, particularly for conditions of nasal inflammation, but it may not feel as comfortable. Warmer water can be used to treat headaches or sinus congestion as it is better for opening the sinuses, but care must be taken so as not to burn the mucus membranes by utilizing such higher temperatures.

Generally beginners should always use only slightly warm water at first. Cooler or warmer water is used more for therapeutic purposes, which we will discuss in the second section of the book.

The Use of Salt in the Neti Pot

The human body does not consist simply of pure water, but of water in which various nutrients, vitamins, minerals and enzymes are held in solution. The basic plasma of the body is a liquid of a slightly oily or viscous nature, reflecting these substances suspended within it. The mucus membranes of the body hold moisture but also have a gelatinous quality.

This means that if we simply flush the mucus membranes with pure water, we can remove this mucus lining and irritate the underlying tissue base. The nose is no different. If we just pour only water through the nose, it can damage the mucus lining. It can also result in pain because the nose has many nerve endings, while many other mucus linings of the body do not.

The main substance in nature that helps us protect this mucus lining is salt, which works in the body to sustain the level of hydration. Our basic plasma itself is an evolution of ocean water, which is salty in nature. *So the use of a little salt is always required in the neti pot to protect the nasal passages.* In Ayurvedic medicine, salt is also used in enemas for the same purpose of protecting the mucus lining.[14]

Non-iodized table salt is best. Iodized salt is more likely to be irritating. Sea salt is also stronger than table salt and sometimes irritating, though some people do use it.

Preparing the Solution for the Neti Pot

Take about 1/4 teaspoon of non-iodized table salt and mix it into about 1 cup of warm water until it dissolves completely. Place approximately half a cup of the solution into the neti pot, which is usually enough to irrigate one of the nostrils.

Note that some people may prefer to add the salt and warm water directly into the neti pot and mix it there. In that case, use about 1/8 teaspoon of salt, depending upon how much water the neti pot can hold. Again make sure to dissolve it completely as undissolved salt can feel irritating to the nose.

However, this amount is only a general guideline; *you can adjust the amount of salt in the solution according to what feels comfortable for you.* More salt may be necessary if the nostrils are drier. Alternatively, you may prefer less salt if you find the salt level to be irritating.

Main Procedure

- Take the filled neti pot to a bathroom sink or a wash basin that can drain away the used water.

- Begin with your right nostril. Tilt your head slightly to the opposite side as shown in the illustration.

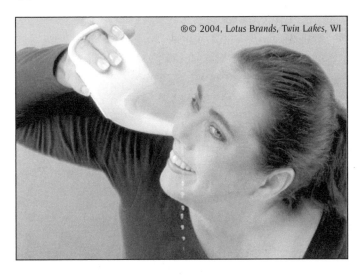

®© 2004, *Lotus Brands, Twin Lakes,* WI

- Insert the spout of the neti pot gently into the raised nostril.

- Slowly pour the water from the neti pot into the nostril until the water filters down, through and out the opposite lower nostril and into the sink.

- Blow through the nostril gently to complete the process and help drain all the water out. Close the other nostril gently with your finger while you are doing this.

Adjustments

- Adjust your head slightly to whatever angle works best for your comfort and for an easy flow of water. Generally placing your forehead at an angle about the same level as your chin works best.

- You can also adjust the flow through the neti pot by raising or lowering the level and tilt of the neti pot itself. The higher you hold it, the faster the water will flow through it.

- While pouring water through the nostrils you will have to breathe through your mouth. Continue breathing in a comfortable manner. There is no need to hold your breath while using the neti pot.

- Some water may not flow easily through the nostrils, but instead may trickle down your nose and face (and beard if you have one). Don't worry about this. Simply let the water flow into the sink.

- The water may come out with some mucus, particularly if you have any congestion or mucus residues in the head. A little mucus discharge is normal. Generally the amount of mucus discharged will decrease through regular usage of the neti pot.

Doing the Opposite Nostril

- Once you have done the right nostril, refill the neti pot and proceed with the left nostril, tilting your head in the opposite direction and otherwise following the same procedures.

Afterwards

- Once you are finished using the neti pot, blow out each of your nostrils gently several times in order to clean them further. More mucus may come out at this point. You can use a handkerchief or paper tissue to catch this.

- You may need to tilt your head from side to side or bend down over the sink to make sure that all the water comes out of your nostrils.

■ Remember that the use of the neti pot should be done slowly and carefully. Never try to force the water through quickly, and never try to blow your nose hard to get it out. Let the water do the work.

Repeating the Procedure

■ If you are so congested that the water doesn't go all the way through, you can try the procedure several times, starting with the nostril that is most open. You will notice that each time you pour the water into the nose it will penetrate further, until eventually it will go all the way through.

■ You can repeat the procedure more than once if mucus or congestion remains, but generally no more than three times. You can wait and try the neti pot again later in the day. You may also try some of the other methods of opening the nostrils that are discussed later in the book in the chapter 'Neti and Ayurvedic Therapies'.

Care of Your Neti Pot

The most important factor to care for the neti pot is to keep it clean. Sometimes a little mucus gets into the neti pot and can adhere to the inside where you may not be able to see it. Regularly clean your neti pot out with hot water and a little soap for this purpose. Make sure to rinse away any soap residues afterwards as these can irritate the nostrils. The "teapot" style ceramic pots are often sturdier than the others and are made to be dishwasher safe to provide effective hot water cleaning of the pot.

It is good to clean or rinse out the neti pot with hot water each time before you use it. After using it, make sure to clean out the sink and surrounding area where any mucus may have been discharged.

Like any other instrument of personal hygiene such as a toothbrush, do not share your neti pot with other people.

If you travel, make sure to pack the neti pot well. Ceramic pots can break. Even at home make sure to place or store your neti pot where it will not be easily knocked over or able to fall on the floor!

Cautions on Using the Neti Pot

While the neti pot is a very safe device, there are some cautions and contraindications that one should be aware of in its usage.

- Do not use the neti pot if there is any significant bleeding from the nostrils. If you have had a nosebleed recently, make sure it has had time to heal properly before using the neti pot.

- Be careful with the neti pot if there is any sinus infection, particularly of an acute nature.

- If your sinuses are completely blocked, also exercise caution. The neti pot can be used in such conditions but requires skill and experience.

- If you are suffering from asthma, be careful using the neti pot during acute attacks.

- If you are a beginner, first master using the neti pot for general health maintenance purposes before using it in a more specific therapeutic matter (such as discussed later in the book).

Dealing with Possible Complications (Troubleshooting)

Below is list of common difficulties or complications that may occur while using the neti pot.

Water from the neti pot drips into my throat and mouth.

Increase the tilt of your head, keeping your chin at the level of the forehead or higher. If only a small amount of water is involved, simply spit out the water. It is no real problem.

Use of the neti results in pain in my nose.

You may need to use a little more or less salt in the water. If you feel a burning sensation, it usually means the salt level is too high. If it is only pain that you feel, the salt level may be too low.

After using the neti pot, my nostrils are not cleared or even become more congested.

Try repeating the procedure, using warmer water, or adding a pinch of a spicy herb like ginger or cinnamon to help open the blockage. Additionally, you may inhale a little of an aromatic oil like menthol or eucalyptus immediately prior to using the neti pot.

If these adjustments do not work, stop using the neti pot. You may need some herbs or medications to clear the blockage first.

Water gets retained in my sinuses and may drip out later, sometimes it makes me feel dull.

If a little water drains out later, don't worry about it. Just use a handkerchief or soft tissue to blow it out.

To prevent water retention, after using the neti pot bend your head or your upper body over, tilting the head from side to side until the water drains out onto the floor. (You might want to put a towel down to catch it and protect the floor, or you can do it over the bathtub or shower floor.)

You can add a pinch of a stimulating, spicy herb to the neti such as calamus or ginger, or inhale a little of an aromatic oil like eucalyptus or menthol. Such practices will aid in removing the water from the sinuses, perhaps even making you sneeze.

If the problem persists, stop using the neti pot. It probably means that you may have some blockages deeper in the sinuses that need to be treated first. Use either a nasya oil with aromatic herbs or inhale the powder of spicy herbs like ginger or cinnamon. Note our section on Ayurvedic therapies for more details on such alternatives to the neti pot when it does not work for you.

After using the neti pot I have to blow my nose repeatedly.

This is often a good sign that your sinuses are opening up. It is seldom a problem. However, remember to always blow your nose gently.

Using the neti pot makes me sneeze.

This is usually not a problem and the sneezing can help clear the nostrils. However, if it happens frequently or often it can be a sign of allergies. Sometimes it occurs if the salt level in the water is too high. You might want to consider reducing the salt a bit and see if it helps. Otherwise you might have to do something additional to treat the allergies.

A little blood comes out along with the water from the neti pot.

A small amount of bleeding may result from not using enough salt in the neti pot. If that is the case, increase the salt level slightly. However, you might want to wait until the membrane heals, as salt can irritate any cut or abrasion.

Bleeding may occur from too much dryness in the nostrils, which causes the membrane to tear. If that is the case, try putting a little sesame oil into the nose prior to using the neti pot, or even into the neti pot (along with the salt). This is more likely to occur in the late spring season when our energy rises along with the increasing outside temperature.

Alternatively, there may be an internal problem in the nostrils. If that is the case, stop using the neti pot and consult a physician to ensure proper treatment.

When to Use the Neti Pot

The use of the neti pot acquires a different relevance at different times of the day or year.

Time of Day

The best time to use the neti pot is early in the morning shortly after one gets up. It should be an integral part of your morning elimination routine, along with scraping the tongue and brushing your teeth.

Since the body is in a prone position during the night mucus accumulates in the head and congestion often develops as a result. It is important to clear this congestion out first thing so that one has a proper flow of energy for the rest of the day.

It is also good to use the neti pot before sleep to ensure that the nasal passages are open for optimal breathing during sleep. This can help prevent snoring and mouth breathing and aid in a deeper and more relaxing sleep.

However, the neti pot can be used any time that one feels congested or blocked in the head and sinuses and wishes to breathe more freely. Even in the absence of any physical discomfort, it can be a beneficial therapy to help a person feel more aware and can aid in clearer thinking.

Seasonal Usage

The neti pot has its usefulness during all seasons.

- In the summer, allergies are more common since there is more abundant pollen in the air. The neti pot can help remove these irritants.

- In the fall, the dryness of the air can irritate the nostrils, causing allergies and other discomfort. This means that one should use more salt or sesame oil in the neti.

- In the winter, coldness and dampness increase and can lodge in the head. This means that we should use warmer water or a little of a spicy herb like calamus or ginger in the neti. We also spend more time indoors during the winter, breathing in more stagnant air and air from heaters that often contains dust. The neti pot helps to counter this.

- Spring time is the natural Kapha season in which mucus can more likely accumulate or flow. The use of the neti will aid in this seasonal discharge. Also during springtime, some people may experience nosebleeds as their energy rises. The neti can help with this.

Usage by Children

Children commonly suffer from sinus congestion and other problems of excess mucus. Childhood is the Kapha phase or formative watery phase of life in Ayurvedic medicine, which is why children often have mucus discharges from the nose.

The neti pot is an excellent remedy for these childhood problems. While it can be difficult for children to learn how to use it initially, an eight to ten year old child can generally learn to do so with a little coaching. But it is best for a responsible adult to be present when children are using the neti pot.

Usage by the Elderly

Many elderly people suffer from dry skin and dryness of the mucus membranes and nostrils, which can impair the breathing process. Old age is the Vata or airy phase of our energy according to Ayurveda, in which the mind continues to grow but the body begins to decline.

The use of the neti pot can help counter such conditions of dryness and debility. The neti pot is a great tool for the elderly who feel lethargic in the morning and can help them get going.

For Women

The neti pot can be safely used during pregnancy, menstruation or menopause. Soothing the flow of energy in the circulatory and nervous systems, it can help indirectly with the pain, blockage or other symptoms that can arise during these times.

The main possible exception is during morning sickness. Some women find that the neti pot can increase nausea if used during that stage of pregnancy. Others are able to use it even during morning sickness and find that it helps calm the symptoms. Ultimately, if you choose to do so at that time, it is advisable to exercise caution in the beginning.

Usage in Special Conditions

For Athletes and Sports Medicine

The neti pot is a great tool to use before any significant physical or athletic exertion for better energy and enhanced performance. It is also a good practice afterwards to soothe the nostrils and clear out any mucus and toxins stirred up by the exertion.

In this way the neti pot is a good aid to anything from running to hiking to weight-lifting, including all competitive sports. It is something for all serious or professional athletes to consider using in order to improve their competitive edge. *The neti pot should be an integral part of any sports medicine.*

When Traveling

When traveling, the sinuses suffer a lot of stress from recycled air, exposure to the air breathed by many people including the possible contagious diseases they may carry and the effects of altitude and possible sleep disruption. While these conditions are most pronounced with air travel, they occur to a lesser degree while traveling by car, train or other modes of transportation.

When traveling, it is good to use the neti pot to help counter these conditions and protect the sinuses from possible problems. It is particularly good to use the neti pot to help deal with the effects of jet lag.

Usage by Those Who Are Ill

Patients who are bedridden easily get sinus congestion or impaired breathing function caused by the long periods of time that they must spend in a prone position. The neti pot can help counter this condition.

Those in convalescence from febrile or infectious diseases often suffer from dryness and dehydration that shows up in dry nasal passages. The neti pot is useful in regard to this condition as well.

Those suffering from chronic lung, sinus or lymphatic problems can benefit from the neti pot for clearing out excess mucus from the body. Those suffering from acute lung or sinus conditions can also benefit from the use of the neti pot but require more care and experience in its usage.

Note the second section of the book for the chapter, Neti and Specific Conditions, for more information on the value of the neti and the process of nasal irrigation in treating many different diseases. But please remember, *if you have any significant health problem that might cause complications, please consult your health care provider before using the neti pot.*

Part II

Advanced Application of the Neti Pot

6.
Neti and Yoga Practices

The neti pot is perhaps the most important device used in classical Yoga. It is the main cleansing method performed preliminary to the practice of Pranayama or yogic breathing exercises. Pranayama emphasizes deep breathing, which first requires that the nostrils are clear, or it will not be fully effective. For this reason, many yogis routinely practice this nasal cleansing at the beginning of any pranayama session. In addition to this, cleansing the nostrils with the neti pot also aids in asana practice, in meditation and with all other yogic methods, for which good circulation of Prana, particularly to the head, is essential.

Neti and Pranayama

Exercising the Nostrils

Probably the most important yogic pranayama practice is 'alternate nostril breathing', where one breathes in exclusively through one nostril and generally out the opposite nostril. This has various names like Nadi Shodhana, Anuloma/Viloma, solar and lunar breathing and other terms in Hatha Yoga.[15]

For this purpose one closes the opposite nostril with the use of light finger pressure and breathes in through the open nostril. *Generally the ring and little fingers of the right hand are used for closing the left nostril and the right thumb for closing the right nostril.* The neti pot, with its emphasis on clearing the nostrils, was mainly devised to facilitate this practice of alternate nostril breathing.

Alternate nostril breathing is probably the best exercise for the nostrils, which as muscles require their proper exertion in order to maintain their tone and flexibility. *Through alternate nostril breathing you can provide a good workout for your nostrils,* which in most of us are weak and otherwise not directly exercised at all. This practice aids in developing the strength of the nostrils, which in turn increases our breathing capacity and vital energy all around.

Weak and blocked nostrils are a primary cause of many ear, nose, throat and lung problems. Strengthening them with alternate nostril breathing is an important means of countering these health problems.

Most of us exercise our arms and legs on a regular basis, without which our bodily strength gets reduced. Yet how many of us consider the proper exercise of our nostrils on which our pranic strength and breathing power depends? Daily alternate nostril breathing is as important to the health of the nose as daily exercise is for the overall health of the body. From a yogic perspective, it is best to remember the neti pot as an aid to alternate nostril breathing.

Solar and Lunar Energy

Our breath usually flows more through one nostril than another at any given moment, switching its current back and forth at different times of the day. This is not simply an incidental event but reflects a fluctuation in our energy, activity and awareness through time, providing important information on what is happening inside ourselves.

In yogic thought the right nostril, along with the right half of the body in general, carries a warming solar energy. It connects to the *Pingala Nadi* or solar pranic current that flows around the spine and its chakra system, energizing the right side of the body. When the breath flows primarily through this nostril, it is good for digestion, circulation, exercise, movement and other more dynamic activities that result from increased heat in the body.

The left nostril, along with the left half of the body in general, carries a cooling lunar energy. It connects to the *Ida nadi* or lunar pranic current, which flows around the spine and its chakra system, and energizes the left side of the body. When the breath flows primarily through this nostril, it is good for relaxation, rest, sleep and the building up of tissue mass and other more soothing actions that depend upon coolness in the body.

Right side breathing develops *Shiva energy*, the cosmic masculine force. Left side breathing develops *Shakti energy*, the cosmic feminine force. In this way alternate nostril breathing has a spiritual effect as well as a physiological action.

Balancing the Right and Left Hemispheres of the Brain

The right and left nostrils and their energy currents relate to the right and left hemispheres of the brain, but in an opposite manner. The right or solar current relates to the left hemisphere of the brain, which, like it, governs rational, perceptive and masculine qualities. The left or lunar current relates to the right hemisphere of the brain, which, like it, governs emotional, receptive and feminine qualities.

The pranic flow through the nostrils has an immediate impact upon the opposite sides of the brain, stimulating their activity. *This means that the combined use of the neti pot and alternate nostril breathing is an ideal exercise for balancing the right and left hemispheres of the brain, helpful for everyone who wants to achieve that balance of mind and emotions.*

Alternate Nostril Breathing and Ayurveda

Relative to Ayurvedic medicine, Pitta dosha as fire relates to the energy of the right, solar Pingala Nadi. When the breath flows through it, digestion, circulation, bodily heat, perception and other Pitta powers get increased. Kapha dosha as water relates to the left, lunar or Ida Nadi. When the breath flows through it, sleep, tissue formation, bodily coolness, emotion and other Kapha powers predominate.

As Ayurvedic treatment is in terms of opposites, for treating Kapha conditions of cold, dampness and mucus, one emphasizes increasing the breath through the right or solar nadi. For treating Pitta conditions of heat and inflammation, one emphasizes increasing the breath through the left or lunar nadi.

Vata dosha, as the biological air humor, results in an erratic flow of breath between the nostrils. So balancing the flow between both nostrils is an important method for calming Vata.

Alternate Nostril Breathing and Self-healing

When one nostril is blocked, then the energy will be inhibited from flowing through that side of the body as a whole, reducing its activities. If the other nostril remains open, then the flow through the corresponding side of the body will be increased, making its activities excessive.

When the left side is blocked and the breath is only flowing in the right nostril, then the person may suffer from insomnia, irritability, hyperactivity and generally more Pitta and Vata problems. When the right side is blocked and the breath is only flowing in the left nostril, then the person may suffer from tiredness, lethargy, poor digestion, poor circulation, dullness of mind and other generally more Kapha and Vata problems.

This means that we can use alternate nostril breathing as a form of self-treatment. If we are feeling tired or fatigued and want to wake up and get more energy, we can perform alternate nostril breathing, emphasizing inhalation through the right nostril. If we are feeling overly stimulated or stressed and want to slow down we can perform alternate nostril breathing emphasizing inhalation through the left nostril.

The neti pot can help us balance the flow of the breath through the two nostrils, even in the absence of pranayama by keeping both nostrils open. *But it is good to perform a few alternate nostril breaths after using the neti pot, ideally up to fifteen minutes worth, to optimize this effect, particularly if we want to use the healing power of the breath.*

Alternate Nostril Breathing and Meditation

Alternate nostril breathing helps open the nostrils to allow for deeper breathing to occur. It also affords us greater control over the flow of the breath. We can draw the air in through each nostril in a measured way, like sucking in water through a straw, while normal breathing through both nostrils at once generally results in a quicker and shallower breathing process.

For this reason, alternate nostril breathing is emphasized in yoga practices, which aim at slowing the breathing process down and holding the breath for longer periods of time. When the breath is held at a deep level, then the fire of the breath rises and helps purify both body and mind.[16]

As mind and breath are related, slowing down the breath also slows down the mind and helps bring us into a quiet, peaceful meditative state. If the breath is calm, the mind is calm. While it is hard to control the mind directly, it is not difficult if one knows how to calm the breath first. All those who practice meditation should remember this important secret of the neti pot and the breath.

Purification of the Nadis

Alternate nostril breathing is the basis of what is called Nadi Shodhana or purification of the nadis in Yogic thought (which is the main Sanskrit term for alternate nostril breathing as well). It helps to purify the subtle channels of the mind and nervous system and open them up to higher flows of energy. These subtler nadis connect to the chakras, therefore clearing them aids in any chakra work as well.

In this regard, alternate nostril breathing is foundational for deeper Yoga practices of Tantra and Kundalini Yoga, the awakening of the higher energy of consciousness within us.

Mantra and Alternate Nostril Breathing

One can use special mantras along with alternate nostril breathing to strengthen its effects. The mantra 'ram' (pronounced with a short vowel sound as in the word the), which holds the subtle energy of fire, can be used along with right nostril breathing to give more power to it. The mantra 'vam' (also pronounced with a short vowel sound as in the word the), which holds the subtle energy of water, can be used along with left-nostril breathing to make it more effective. For retention one can mentally recite the mantra Om in the same manner.

One should develop a rhythm with the mantra according to the length of one's breath. In the beginning a good ratio is eight beats per inhalation, eight per retention and eight per exhalation. For right nostril breathing one can mentally recite the mantra ram eight times during inhalation via the right nostril and the mantra vam eight times during exhalation through the left nostril. Eventually one can prolong the exhalation to twice that of the inhalation. More advanced yogis will retain the breath after exhalation as well, but such practices are best done following direct instruction from a teacher.

Neti and Asana Practice

Asanas that bring the energy into the head and sinuses can sometimes result in sinus blockages by moving mucus into the region. This includes headstand, shoulderstand and other inverted postures. For those who wish to do such asanas, the use of the neti pot can be an important aid.

It is helpful to use the neti pot prior to any asana practice in order to open the head, promote deeper breathing and cleanse the deeper channels. It can similarly be good to use the neti pot after asana practice if one feels any blockage or pressure in the head as a result of practice, or just to aid in the detoxification process, which asanas promote. This includes not only asanas that affect the head, but also those that work on the lungs and other sites of mucus accumulation.

The Six Cleansing Methods of Hatha Yoga

Classical Hatha Yoga emphasizes six methods (shat-karma) of internal cleansing, of which neti or nasal cleansing is one.[17] These are important methods of removing toxins from the body.

1. **Cleansing the Stomach (Dhauti)**

   This was done traditionally through the use of a special cloth that the yogi swallowed for this purpose, which requires skill and training. The same result on a safer level can occur through the use of expectorant (mucus-expelling) herbs and therapies, and therapeutic vomiting (vamana in Ayurvedic parlance), which is the main Ayurvedic method of reducing excess Kapha that accumulates in the stomach as phlegm.

2. **Cleansing the Colon (Vasti or Basti)**

   This was done mainly with the use of water and herbal enemas. It is also an important Ayurvedic practice for eliminating excess Vata dosha, which accumulates in the colon as gas and fecal matter. For this purpose, Ayurveda has an entire set of special enema formulas and practices.

3. **Cleansing the Nostrils (Neti)**

   This traditionally had two forms. The first was using a cloth (Sutra Neti), which like Dhauti requires skill and guidance and should not be attempted on one's own. The second is water cleansing (Jala Neti) or the use of the Neti pot that we have outlined in this book. This is an important Ayurvedic method for eliminating the doshas or toxins from the head, the foremost of which is Kapha dosha or excess mucus.

4. **Cleansing the Eyes (Trataka)**

   This involves focusing the eyes steadily until tears arise. The use of herbs like a little onion juice into the eyes is another way of doing this. Trataka not only strengthens the eyes but also helps remove any doshas from them, particularly Pitta, which relates to the eyes.

5. **Stimulating the Digestive Fire or Agni (Nauli)**

   In traditional Hatha Yoga, this is done with special muscular movements and contractions in the navel area. It can also be promoted internally through taking various digestion-promoting herbs and spices like ginger, cayenne and black pepper.[18] Stimulating Agni is a central Ayurvedic therapy because all doshic derangements, whether of Vata, Pitta or Kapha, usually either cause or result in digestive system or Agni impairments.

6. **Kapalabhati, Strong Pranayama or Rapid Deep Breathing**

   This is a pranayama technique of rapid inhalation and exhalation, done like the bellows of a blacksmith. It is also very powerful for opening the sinuses and lungs. It is another important method for reducing Kapha dosha or excess mucus from the body. Kapalabhati is another good breathing exercise to do after using the neti pot, just as the use of the neti pot is a good preliminary practice for it.

These six yogic methods can be related to many of the detoxification methods that are popular in natural healing today. Of the six, the use of the neti pot is probably the easiest to do. To practice Yoga effectively, yogic texts recommend that any disease causing toxins or doshas should first be removed by such cleansing practices. Ayurvedic medicine uses similar practices in its Pancha-Karma detoxification system of radical cleansing, which employs enemas, therapeutic vomiting and various nasal methods. Such detoxification measures are the necessary foundation for any rebuilding or rejuvenative practices.

7.
Neti and Ayurvedic Therapies

Ayurvedic medicine contains an entire range of health therapies, which aim at treating the nose, sinuses and related regions of the head and throat. These are called 'nasya' therapies, or 'what relates to the nose,' or *nasa* in Sanskrit. We can compare these with ear, nose and throat therapies in modern medicine, but they are also used along with other treatment methods for health problems for both body and mind.

The neti pot is an important tool of nasya therapies. Other nasya methods involve placing medicated oils into the nose with eyedroppers, snuffing powdered herbs, massage of the nasal region and other forms of steam therapy and massage to the head. The use of the neti pot can be enhanced by these other nasya methods and can be used along with them.

The Neti Pot and the Doshas

Each of the three doshas of Vata, Pitta and Kapha can benefit from nasya and neti therapies in its own way. Following I have listed these main factors.

The Neti Pot and the Treatment of Kapha

Kapha as mucus accumulates in the upper portion of the body from the stomach, where most of it originates according to Ayurveda, to the lungs, where it overflows, to the head, where it blocks up.

Because of their value in dispelling mucus, nasya and neti therapies are primary methods for treating Kapha disorders and removing Kapha excesses. They should be considered for all Kapha diseases and should form an integral part of a healthy life-style for all Kapha types.

All Kapha types should practice nasya and neti on a regular basis as an aid to keep Kapha in check and maintain positive health and vitality. This is particularly important when signs of high Kapha in the body occur like swollen lymph glands, coughing of mucus, congestion and low energy.

Kapha-type diseases include colds, flu, allergies, asthma and other diseases of excess mucus. They extend to arthritis, diabetes and coronary heart disease. Another important Kapha condition is obesity or being overweight. Excess Kapha results in excess tissue formation, particularly of the adipose or fat tissue.

High Kapha in the head dulls the mind and senses and reduces our capacity for concentration. It makes us more sedentary in our activity, reducing our overall functional activity. It results in oversleeping, which in turn increases Kapha further.

By stimulating the movement and elimination of excess Kapha dosha, nasya and neti help treat all such Kapha conditions.

The Neti Pot and the Treatment of Vata

Vata dosha, as composed of air and ether elements, is the prime dosha relating to Prana or the vital force. When the sinuses are blocked, Prana, the positive energy of Vata dosha, is also blocked, impairing our overall energy production and circulation. This prevents the positive energy of Vata from developing as creativity, curiosity, motivation and enthusiasm. For promoting the positive aspect of Vata dosha, neti and nasya are primary therapies.

Vata diseases include diseases of Vata systems of the bones, excretory system, nervous system and mind. Nasya and neti are important treatment measures for such Vata conditions. They help restore the organic equilibrium of the mind and body and our hormonal secretions that are ruled by Prana. They are important considerations for Vata diseases, particularly those involving the mind and brain.

The Neti Pot and the Treatment of Pitta

Pitta dosha, like fire, tends to rise upward, bringing heat, inflammation and tension to the head and eyes. Pitta energy from the liver and small intestine, its main sites of production, frequently moves in this direction.[19] This may result in anything from a minor energy influx to more serious conditions like hypertension and stroke. Emotionally, it can increase anger and irritability and make a person hot-headed.

Pitta diseases include most diseases of the blood, including many inflammatory and infectious conditions in the body. Keeping the energy in the head clear and cool through nasya and neti therapies can help alleviate all such conditions. They can protect the eyes and help promote our vision.

Use of Herbs and Oils in the Neti Pot

The neti pot is an instrument through which not only water, but also herbs and oils can be applied to the nose. Many of us may find the idea of pouring herbal decoctions through our nostrils to be strange, but note that the mucus lining of the nose does have an absorptive capacity, so it can also extract the healing energy from the herbs.

An important Ayurvedic principle is to treat a condition both locally at the site as well as systemically through the body as a whole. For example, if you have a wound or a sore you will place an ointment or salve directly upon it, as well as take anti-infection medications internally. For treating the colon, you would likely use an enema, not just take a purgative. Thus for treating the sinuses and head a direct application of herbs through the nostrils is a good strategy. The herbs can have a more powerful and immediate effect at the site of the problem than if they are simply consumed as an herbal tea or taken as a pill.

The nasal cavity is an important opening for a broad range of herbal therapies. The nostrils are an important site for treating all disorders of the head, ear, nose and throat, as well as all conditions involving the mind and emotions. Not surprisingly, some form of nasya therapy is often recommended for most Ayurvedic patients.

Though the basic use of the neti pot only involves salt, one can add other therapeutic substances to it. The neti pot is a particularly important vehicle for using nervine herbs, including both stimulants and sedatives. When we apply them through the nose the herbs can have a stronger affect upon the brain.

Adding Oils to the Neti Pot

If the nostrils are dry, one can add a few drops of a natural oil to the neti pot solution in order to help lubricate the nostrils and protect the mucus membranes. The most common such oil used is sesame, which has special nutritive and anti-pain properties as well as the greatest power of penetration of all natural oils. Other oils like almond, apricot, coconut or olive can be used in the same manner.

For this purpose add ½ teaspoon of a natural oil like sesame to the neti solution and stir it gently before pouring it into the nostril.

However, if you do this, make sure to avoid getting oil on your clothes or on the floor. The use of oils in the neti pot requires that we are more careful while using it and cleaning up afterwards.

Many people find it easier to apply the oil directly to the nostrils through an eyedropper first and then use the neti pot in the usual way without oil later. We will note this practice later in this chapter under 'Nasya Oils'.

For more complex treatments, natural oils and herbs can be used together in the neti pot. In this case one should cook the oil along with the herbs for a few minutes so that their properties get mixed together and then add them to the neti solution.

How to Prepare Herbs for the Neti Pot

The simplest method is to make a warm infusion of the herbs first, steeping the herbs in hot water similar to making tea, and adding the resultant herbal tea to the water for the neti pot.

However, care must be taken that the infusion, particularly of spicy herbs, is not too strong. Start with a weak infusion like ¼ teaspoon of the herb per cup of water.

You can always increase the strength as needed, or just use some warm water from an herbal tea diluted into the water for the neti pot.

A second and simpler method is to add a few pinches of the powdered herb directly to the warm water for the neti pot, allowing it a few moments to soak. However, make sure that the particles of the herbs are not so large so as to irritate the nose and make you sneeze or cause other discomfort. Filter the mixture first if this might be a problem.

A third method is to take a few leaves of an aromatic herb like mint, sage or basil and soak it in a cup of cool or lukewarm water over night, preferably in a copper vessel. This is a cold infusion in western herbal parlance. Use this water in the morning for the neti pot solution, but warm it up a little first.

Cleansing or Tonifying Therapies

Ayurvedic therapies are broadly divided into two main groups as either cleansing or tonifying. Cleansing therapies aim at removing toxins and reducing excesses, particularly accumulations of Vata, Pitta and Kapha. Most usage of the neti pot occurs on this level and can be enhanced by other detoxifying nasal (nasya) therapies.

Tonifying therapies aim at either building bodily tissues or at increasing overall vitality, including fortifying the immune system. The neti pot can be used in this way as well. This requires the addition of tonifying herbs and oils to the usual salt mixture.

Generally the use of cleansing therapies precedes that of tonifying therapies, as one must remove toxins first before rebuilding.

1. Cleansing Therapies and the Neti Pot

To aid in cleansing the nostrils and sinuses various herbs, mainly spicy in taste, are added to the neti mixture. Many of these spices have nervine properties to stimulate the brain and senses and can help counter dullness, depression and mental fatigue. Many are expectorants, which are herbs good for removing mucus and diaphoretics, or herbs that promote sweating and improve peripheral circulation, including circulation to the head.

Mild Spices and Aromatics

The best herbs to use as cleansing agents in the neti pot are mild spices. These include sage, thyme, basil, spearmint and peppermint. Other pungent tasting mucus-reducing herbs like elecampane or bayberry can be used in the same manner.

Tulsi or Indian Holy Basil

Tulsi (*Ocinum sanctum*) or Indian Holy Basil is one of the best herbs for the brain, nerves and heart and is perhaps the best herb to use in the neti pot. It is traditionally used in the practice of Yoga for promoting devotion and for awakening higher perceptual capacities. It is excellent for colds, flu, allergies and sinus problems.

Ginger

Ginger is probably the most common herb for Ayurvedic nasya therapy. Ginger is particularly effective for opening the sinuses, stimulating the senses and promoting the perceptive activity of the brain.

However, ginger is warming, if not hot, and can be irritating in its effects. Use it first in low dosages, either a few pinches of the powder or a weak infusion. Don't be surprised if it makes you sneeze or blow your nose. This can be a good sign that it is working to clear out the nostrils and sinuses.

Another good spice for this purpose is cinnamon. Cardamom can also be used but only in a mild solution. Nutmeg can help promote sleep.

Calamus

Traditional Ayurveda mainly uses the herb calamus (*Acorus calamus*) for cleansing the sinuses and adds it to many nasya oils. A few pinches of calamus powder can be added to the neti for this purpose, or a mild infusion can be made and the water added to the mixture. Calamus is particularly effective for opening the sinuses, stimulating the senses and promoting the perceptive activity of the brain. It is often used post-stroke to bring back the power of speech and revitalize the nerves.

However, note that the FDA does not recommend calamus for internal consumption as an herbal tea. Its usage in the neti mixture, however, is not a problem.

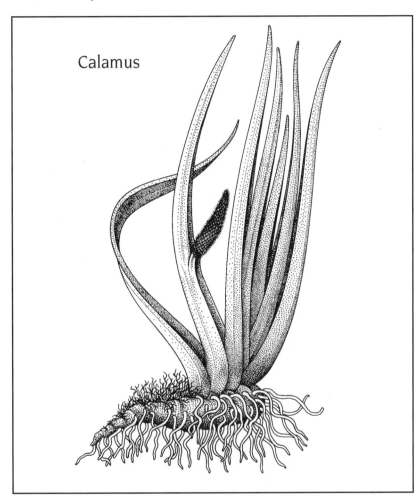

Calamus

Cooling Herbs

Besides spicy herbs, which are used mainly for their warming action, bitter and astringent herbs, which have a cooling nature, can be added for reducing heat and inflammation in the head and for promoting healing of the nasal passages. Some of these bitters have nervine properties to open, clear and calm the mind and senses. Good herbs of this type include skullcap, hops and lady's slipper.

While most spices are heating, some like spearmint and coriander have mild cooling effects as well and can be employed for such conditions.

Even stronger nervine sedatives like valerian or its Ayurvedic relative jatamamsi (Nardostachys jatamansi)[20] can be used in this way, but their taste and smell can be unpleasant, which may be difficult for many people to handle in their nostrils!

Gotu Kola and Brahmi

Gotu kola is probably the best herb for this purpose, combining nervine, astringent and bitter properties. A few pinches of gotu kola powder can be added to the neti solution or an infusion of the herb. Gotu kola herb has a cooling, calming and clearing effect upon the mind and senses.

A close Ayurvedic relative named Brahmi (Hydrocotyle asiatica) is actually a little better but not always available at regular herb stores. It is considered to have rejuvenative (rasayana) effects for improving memory, promoting meditation and countering the aging process. Taken in the neti pot it can have a much stronger and more immediate effect upon the brain. Manduka parni (Bacopa monnieri) is another Ayurvedic herb and Brahmi substitute that can be used as well.[21]

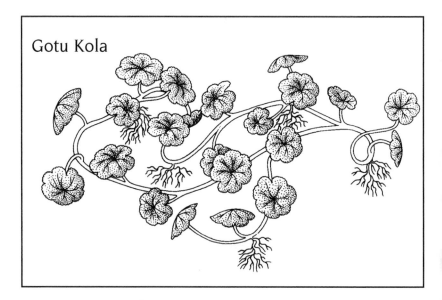

Gotu Kola

Sandalwood

A very mild cold infusion of sandalwood (not the oil but the wood or powder) is very good for its cooling action. It can be added to the neti mixture for calming the mind, nerves and heart and for reducing fever, inflammation or heat in the head.

2. Tonifying Therapies and the Neti Pot

For individuals suffering from dryness of the nostrils and deficiency of weight or bodily fluids, a tonifying approach is indicated. For this purpose, one adds a little of a nutritive oil like sesame to the nasya mixture, as already mentioned, or simply applies the oil directly into the nostrils.

Another method is to add a demulcent herb (one that soothes the mucus membranes) to the neti mixture. Probably, the best herb for this purpose is licorice but it should be used in a light infusion, which is very soothing to the nose and throat. Other demulcent herbs like slippery elm, marshmallow, comfrey root or the Ayurvedic herb shatavari (*Asparagus racemosa*) can be used in such light infusions as well. They can help loosen dry mucus in the head and aid in its liquefaction and removal from the body.

Ayurvedic Nasya Oils

The most important method of nasya or nasal therapy in Ayurvedic medicine is the use of oils like sesame, either by themselves or along with various herbs. We have already discussed adding small amounts of sesame and other oils in the neti pot. These oils can also be placed directly into the nose with the help of an eyedropper, or they can be rubbed lightly into the nostrils by putting a few drops on your little finger.

Placing a few drops of sesame oil into the nostrils helps remove dryness and soothe pain and irritation. However, it can increase congestion. If that is a problem, such oils are not used unless aromatic herbs are added to them to counter this effect.

For nasya therapy Ayurveda mainly uses various 'medicated sesame oils' (Siddha tailas), herbs that are prepared or cooked in a sesame oil base. There are several special Nasya Oils prepared by various Ayurvedic companies, pharmacies or clinics that are now available on the market.

For cleansing the nostrils, spicy and aromatic herbs like camphor, eucalyptus, mint, calamus and ginger are used in the oil base. For soothing and tonifying the nostrils, demulcent herbs like licorice or shatavari are used as cooked in the oil base, like the traditional formula Anu Taila.

Such oil therapy, called *snehana* in Ayurveda, is an important Ayurvedic therapy, particularly for dealing with Vata or high air conditions.

Nasya Oils and the Neti Pot

Nasya oils can be used even more simply and readily than the neti pot. When one needs to treat the nostrils at any time of the day, one just places a few drops of the oil into them. Some oil may come out or cause one to sneeze or clear the nostrils, but you can use a tissue or handkerchief to easily handle this. It is particularly good to take a nasya oil with you when you travel. You can use it on the plane or in the airport when the neti pot is inconvenient.

People who have congestion often do better using an aromatic nasya oil preparation rather than the neti pot. Those who have a lot of dryness in their nostrils will do well using a soothing nasya preparation or simply placing sesame oil into the nose. It is also good to apply a nasya oil after using the neti pot in order to strengthen and prolong its effects.

Whenever you think of the neti pot and its usage, remember the use of nasya oils as well. The two are related therapies and work well together.

One can purchase various types of nasya oils from different Ayurvedic companies and clinics. Often one's Ayurvedic therapist will prescribe it and carry it. It will usually be a small bottle of the oil with an eyedropper.

Neti and Other Therapies

Aroma Therapy

The use of spicy and aromatic herbs in the neti pot solution is itself a kind of aroma therapy. Aromatic herbs have a powerful action to open the nostrils and sinuses. However, one should never use the essential or aromatic oils of herbs directly in the neti because essential oils can be powerful irritants and even burn and damage the mucus membrane, even the oils of cooling herbs like sandalwood. Use a mild infusion of the cut, sifted or powdered herbs instead.

A related aroma therapy is to apply a small amount of an aromatic oil at the base of the nose where one can easily inhale it throughout the day. In this way you can use aromatic oils like camphor, eucalyptus, mint or wintergreen.

It is good to inhale a little of such an aromatic oil after using the neti pot to help open the sinuses further. One can leave a drop or two of the oil at the base of the nostrils to increase the effect of the neti pot afterwards. Natural pain balms like Tiger Balm or Ayurvedic pain oils, which contain such aromatic herbs, can be used in the same way.

Steam Therapy and the Use of Hot Compresses

Another important nasya therapy is placing a hot compress on the region of the nostrils and sinuses. A small amount of a spicy aromatic oil like eucalyptus or wintergreen, or a little ginger powder can be added to the compress in order to heighten the effect. This can be done prior to the use of the neti pot for those requiring something stronger to open the sinuses, or it can be used as a substitute for the neti pot. It is particularly good for those suffering from sinus headaches.

Inhaling steam, particularly that from aromatic herbs like ginger, mint or eucalyptus, is another method. Aromatic oils can be added to water for the steam in small amounts or small amounts of aromatic herbs can be cooked in it. However, be careful because such aromatic oils can irritate the face and cause redness (you can guard against this by placing a little sesame oil or coconut oil on your face).

Ayurveda contains many such steam therapies called *swedana*, which is an important detoxification therapy used on many levels.

Facial Massage and Marma Therapy

Facial massage is a good practice to do before the use of the neti pot, particularly in situations of congestion or to aid in clearing the sinuses as a whole. In this regard Ayurvedic medicine recommends the manipulation of certain energy points on the body called *marmas*, which roughly resemble acupuncture points.

Phana marma or the 'serpent point' is the marma region by the nostrils. The main Phana marma point, which is about as big as the tip of your finger, is located at the outside base of the nostrils at the bottom of the nose. Secondary points exist along the side of the nose up to where the bone connects to the nasal cartilage. One can apply acupressure to these points or massage them in a gentle circular or up and down manner.

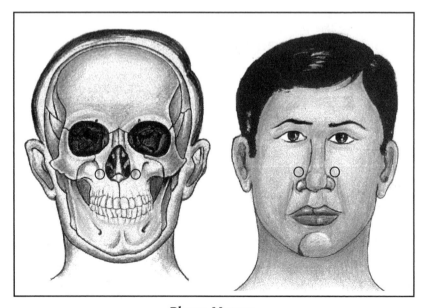

Phana Marma

It is good to massage the entire outer perimeter of the nasal bone, from the bottom to the top of the nose, gently pressing the soft cartilage of the nose as well. If you do this on yourself, you can use the middle fingers of your hands and do both sides of the nostrils simultaneously, working your way from the bottom to the top of the nose and down again applying a gentle but firm pressure and an up and down motion, holding the pressure for a time with a circular motion at any sensitive areas that you may encounter along the way.

Another good area to massage along with using the neti is the region below the cheekbone near the upper margin of the teeth and jaw. This connects to the soft palate and helps open the sinuses internally. It is the area of *Shringataka marma* in Ayurvedic thought and connects to the soft palate and interior sinuses. For self-massage you can continue from the bottom of the nose down and out to this point beneath the upper jawbone and hold the pressure there for some time to open up the energy.

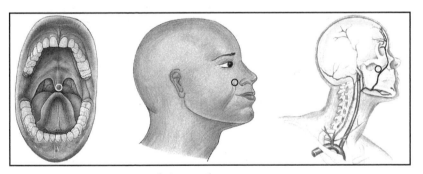

Shringataka Marma

Other special marma points around the eyes like A*panga Marma* at the outside corner of the eye sockets can aid in drainage of mucus from the sinuses behind the eyes and help treat sinus headaches.[22]

Gargling of Herbs

Gargling of herbs or rinsing of the throat is another helpful adjunct to the use of the neti pot and all nasal therapies that target the nose. For additional cleansing action on the head and throat, one can gargle with a little salt or special herbs like turmeric[23] or bayberry or other mild spices and astringents.

Gargling is good not only for sore throats but for any throat irritation, laryngitis or dry throat conditions in general (use oils like sesame or demulcent herbs like licorice for such dryness problems).

Such cleansing of the throat aids in the discharge of mucus from the sinuses. It is good to do when the nostrils are too blocked to use the neti pot. It can help open them to allow one to subsequently use the neti pot.

Eye Washes

Ayurveda has an entire set of eyewashes as well (called *netra basti*). Simple cool water can be used as well as mild herbal mixtures like rose water may be poured or dropped gently into the eyes. In western herbalism, herbs like eyebright or chrysanthemum flowers are specific for this purpose.

However, be very careful not to place any spicy or warming herbs or herbal oils into the eyes, as these can be powerful eye irritants. No herbal essential oils should be used, including sandalwood, as these can irritate the eye as well.

A little sesame oil or ghee (clarified butter) can be used to soothe the eyes, either placed directly in the eyes or simply put on the eyelids and the region around the eyes. Ghee is actually preferable in this instance as it has a special affinity with the eyes.

Such cleansing and soothing of the eyes can be a good adjunct to the neti pot and other nasya therapies. It is great for treating eye problems and helping to drain the sinuses behind the eyes.

8.
Neti and Specific Conditions

The use of the neti pot can help with many health problems, but usually requires the guidance of a health care professional if one wants to use special herbs and oils in the neti solution.

Following I have listed a number of important conditions that the neti pot and related nasya therapies can be especially useful for. Such methods will not necessarily cure these conditions but can aid in reducing the symptoms involved and are worthy of inclusion among their different types of treatment. Please examine Ayurvedic treatment books for details on how to approach such health complaints from a yogic perspective.[24]

Deviated Septum

Many people are born with a deviated septum, which inhibits the airflow through one nostril or the other. Often one nostril may be more than seventy percent blocked all the time. Naturally that nostril will tend more to congestion, which can lead to other health problems and a general energy imbalance in the body.

Use of the neti pot is particularly important for keeping both nostrils open when this is the case. If the deviation is minor, regular use of the neti pot can be a good substitute for corrective surgery, which may have side effects.

Nasal Polyps

The neti pot can help correct nasal polyps by soothing the mucus lining of the nose and improving circulation in the region. More specific herbs can aid in this purpose, depending upon the nature and the cause of the polyps, including herbs that have the power to reduce them. [25]

Colds and Flu

The use of the neti pot, particularly along with spicy herbs like ginger in small amounts, is a good therapy for treating mild colds and flu. It is great for the congestion of an initial head cold, as long as it is not too severe. Remember to use the neti pot along with taking herbal teas like ginger and cinnamon.

The neti pot can also aid in the treatment of coughs, especially those that result from the dripping of mucus from the head into the throat, whether chronic or acute.

Swollen Glands

By removing mucus from the head and opening up the circulation of energy, the use of the neti pot can help cleanse the entire lymphatic system and reduce swollen glands, particularly those in the head, neck and chest regions. It can help with enlarged adenoids in children.

Sinus Allergies

The use of the neti pot is one of the best therapies for sinus allergies of all types. It is best during the non-acute phase of the disease as a preventative measure. It can be used in the acute phase but requires more expertise.

If the nostrils are kept clear, the body is able to filter out the pollen and pollutants that cause or aggravate the allergies. If your allergy season is coming shortly, you should consider preparing yourself for it by regular use of the neti pot. If your allergy season is upon you, remember to use the neti pot to protect you from pollen.

Asthma

For patients suffering from asthma, particularly owing to allergies, it is important to keep the nasal passages clear of allergens, irritants and pollutants. The neti pot is great for doing this. It is worth considering as an integral part of any asthmatic's daily regimen, though it is no substitute for the usual methods of treatment.

Headaches

The neti pot is a good preventative measure for sinus headaches. Some people find it helpful in dealing with migraines and other types of headache as well. Improving circulation in the head, its effects can extend to many types of head pain or discomfort. The use of herbs like ginger or calamus in or along with the neti pot can provide additional relief.

Poor Digestion

According to Ayurvedic and yogic thought, Prana or the vital energy behind the breath is also the basis of the digestive fire and is itself the power that allows us to eat our food. This means if our pranic force is weak, our appetite and digestion are likely to be impaired.

Improving our power of breath or Prana can be a helpful aid for improving digestion. Anyone suffering from digestive problems should consider the neti pot as an additional aid, particularly if they also suffer from a diminished breathing capacity.

Accumulation of mucus in the head is related to the accumulation of toxins in the digestive tract.[26] Mucus in the head often occurs along with mucus in the digestive tract and is mirrored by a thick, greasy tongue coating. If you have both a coating on your tongue and congestion in the nostrils, the two conditions may be part of the same problem. Treating one can help treat the other.

Constipation

The lungs and large intestine are connected in their function according to both Chinese and Ayurvedic systems of medicine. This means that if our nostrils are blocked, there may be a corresponding dysfunction or sluggishness in the colon. If this is the case, the use of the neti pot can aid in promoting elimination as well.

Obesity

The relevance of the neti pot in the treatment of obesity and overweight has already been noted earlier in the book. Daily usage of the neti pot stimulates digestion and circulation and helps promote the removal of mucus, water and excess fat from the body.

Particularly good is using the neti pot along with a small amount of stimulating herbs like ginger, cinnamon or calamus, which promote the burning up of fat in the body. While not a direct method of weight reduction, the use of the neti pot can be a good secondary aid.

Skin Diseases/Acne

The use of the neti pot helps promote circulation, which can help in dealing with skin conditions, rashes or growths, particularly those that occur in the region of the head, face or neck.

Excess mucus is also a common cause of acne. By promoting the discharge of mucus, the neti pot can help with this condition as well. As dry skin on the head is connected with dry nostrils, the use of the neti pot and soothing nasya oils can help with that problem as well.

Arthritis

Arthritis is a disease of poor circulation and the accumulation of toxins in the bones. The use of the neti pot stimulates the flow of Prana through the nervous system and circulation through the skeletal system as well. Therefore, while not a primary therapy for arthritis, the neti pot can still be a useful aid.

Heart Disease

The use of the neti pot can aid in promoting circulation and removal of mucus and plaque (which is a form of mucus) from the respiratory and circulatory systems. In this way it can be a helpful support measure for heart patients, particularly when practiced along with deep breathing (pranayama).[27]

Since in yogic thought the mind and heart are connected, we should also consider other yogic methods such as meditation for such conditions as well.

Insomnia

Insomnia can be related to blockage of the sinuses. The resultant poor breathing prevents deep sleep. If this is the case, using the neti pot before sleep can be an important aid. But it must be used for at least a month to have its full effect. It is not a quick remedy.

Some insomnia is associated with sleep apnea, or failure to breathe that results in palpitations, which wake the person. The neti pot can help prevent this condition as well.

Snoring is another sleep related problem that the use of the neti pot can help correct. If the nostrils are clear, snoring, which consists of breathing through the mouth, is less likely to occur.

Weak Immune Function

By strengthening the breath and the vital force in general, protecting our nostrils and guarding against their vulnerability to the outside pathogens, the neti pot is helpful for any low immune conditions. The practice of pranayama, or yogic breathing, is yet a more important tool of raising our immune response capacity.

Anyone suffering from low immune function, whether mild or severe, should consider such Yogic and Ayurvedic therapies at least as lifestyle support measures.[28]

Chronic Fatigue/Low Energy

Most chronic fatigue syndrome and many related low energy conditions are associated with poor breathing and blocked sinuses. The regular use of the neti pot and pranayama can be important aids in their treatment as well. More Prana always means more energy, which helps us on all levels.

Convalescence

We have already noted that the neti pot is good for convalescent and bedridden patients who cannot exercise much, get sluggish and easily accumulate mucus in the head. However, the use of the neti pot can aid in recovery from almost any disease, helping to restore the vital energy within us. This is particularly true of diseases of the head, lungs and heart.

Nervous System Disorders

By improving the circulation in the head, brain and nervous system, use of the neti pot helps in a general way for all nervous system disorders.

It is particularly good for post-stroke patients. It helps them to regain their faculties such as speech because of its stimulation, not only of the nerves but also of our sensory and motor organs. Because it improves circulation to the head the neti pot can help with shingles, TMJ and other nerve pain conditions in the head.

Psychological Disorders

Just as with nervous system conditions, by improving circulation through the brain and nervous system the use of the neti pot helps with psychological problems. It is particularly good for dullness, depression and anxiety, which are related to poor circulation in the head. It is hard to think clearly, be calm and happy, or deal with stress if our sinuses are blocked and our breathing is impaired.

Other yogic methods like mantra and meditation are very helpful for psychological conditions and should be considered as well.

Depression

Emotional depression is often linked to, or caused by, poor energy circulation in the brain and senses. The neti pot can be an important tool to treat this. It is certainly easier to use and less expensive than the many anti-depression drugs flooding the market today. It is prudent to check your nostrils first to determine if difficulty breathing through them is part of your condition.

Anxiety

Anxiety is often connected to a feeling of difficulty in breathing, or from breathing through the mouth. Using the neti pot to facilitate better breathing might help with this condition as well. Note your breathing pattern if you are feeling anxiety and see if this is the case.

Conclusion

While the neti pot is not a panacea, there are few health problems that its regular usage cannot help to improve. And, of course, it is always a useful tool for disease prevention and promoting greater health, vitality and awareness. The neti pot can reduce the need for antibiotics and other sinus medications and save us from unnecessary visits to the doctor. It is a wonderful tool to help us take control of our own health, aiding us in the deep breathing that can transform our lives.

Remember, such simple methods that you use to improve your own health have long term benefits that can be as important as complex therapies and detailed medical procedures. May the use of this little device bring you better health, energy and awareness!

Part III

Appendices and Resources

1.
Glossary of Terms

Agni—Digestive Fire

Alternate Nostril Breathing—A yogic breathing practice in which we breathe through one nostril at a time while keeping the other nostril closed.

Asana—Yoga posture

Ayurveda—Traditional Indian or Yogic Medicine.

Chakras—Subtle energy centers.

Doshas—Biological humors of Ayurveda.

Hatha Yoga—The main yoga system for working on the physical body.

Ida—Left nostril channel, lunar in nature.

Kapha—Biological water humor.

Kundalini—Subtle energy of higher Yoga practices.

Mantra—Healing sound energy.

Marmas—Ayurvedic energy and pressure points.

Nadi—Subtle channel of the mind, prana or nervous system.

Nadi Shodhana—Purification of the channels or nadis. Another name for alternate nostril breathing.

Nasal irrigation—Cleaning the nostrils by pouring water through them.

Nasa—Nose

Nasya—Nasal therapies of Ayurvedic medicine.

Nasya oil—Ayurvedic medicated oils that are placed in the nostrils, generally with the help of an eyedropper. They are usually prepared with a sesame oil base to which various herbs and spices are added.

Neti—The process of cleansing the nostrils, generally through the use of water.

Neti pot—Small water pot for nasal irrigation.

Pancha Karma—Ayurvedic five-fold detoxification system including the use of enemas, purgatives, therapeutic vomiting, nasal therapies and therapeutic release of toxic blood.

Pingala—Right nostril channel, solar in nature.

Pitta—Biological fire humor.

Prana—Life-force, vital energy, power of the breath.

Pranayama—Yogic breathing and energy practices.

Snehana—Ayurvedic oil therapy.

Swedana—Ayurvedic steam therapy.

Taila—Ayurvedic medicated oil.

Tonification therapy—Therapy for increasing body weight, strength and vitality.

Tulsi—Holy basil, an important Ayurvedic nasya herb.

Vata—Biological air humor.

Vayu—Cosmic air element and universal life-force.

Yoga—System for uniting the individual with the greater universal consciousness.

2.
Bibliography

Chopra, Deepak and David Simon. *The Seven Spiritual Laws of Yoga*. Hoboken, New Jersey: John Wiley and Sons, Inc. 2004.

Frawley, Ranade and Lele. *Ayurveda and Marma Therapy: Energy Points in Yogic Healing*. Twin Lakes, Wisconsin: Lotus Press, 2003.

Frawley, Dr. David. *Ayurvedic Healing: A Comprehensive Guide*, second edition. Twin Lakes, Wisconsin: Lotus Press, 2001.

Frawley. Dr. David. *Yoga and Ayurveda: Self-Healing and Self-Realization*. Twin Lakes, Wisconsin: Lotus Press, 1999.

Frawley and Kozak. *Yoga for Your Type: An Ayurvedic Guide to Your Asana Practice*. Twin Lakes, Wisconsin: Lotus Press, 2001.

Frawley, Dr. David and Dr. Vasant Lad. *The Yoga of Herbs*. Twin Lakes, Wisconsin: Lotus Press, 1986.

Hatha Yoga Pradipika of Svatmarama.

Iyengar, B.K.S. *Light on Pranayama*. New York, NY: Crossroad, 1998.

Joshi, Dr. Sunil. *Ayurveda and Panchakarma*. Twin Lakes, Wisconsin: Lotus Press, 1997.

Lad, Dr. Vasant. *Ayurveda, The Science of Self-Healing*. Twin Lakes, Wisconsin: Lotus Press, 1984.

Rama, Swami, Dr. R. Ballentine and Dr. A. Hymes. *Science of Breath*. Honesdale, PA: Himalayan Institute Press, 1998.

Shivananda, Swami. *The Science of Pranayama*. Tehri-Garhwal, India: Divine Life Society, 1978.

Vishnudevananda. *Complete Illustrated Book of Yoga.*

Smith, Atreya. *Prana, The Secret of Yogic Healing.* York Beach, Maine: Samuel Weiser, 1996.

Yoga Sutras of Patanjali.

3.
Resources

Ayurveda Centers and Training

American Institute of Vedic Studies
Dr. David Frawley (Pandit Vamadeva Shastri), Director
PO Box 8357
Santa Fe, NM 87504-8357
Ph: 505-983-9385
Fax: 505-982-9156
Email: vedicinst@aol.com
Website: www.vedanet.com

Aryavaidya Shala (Coimbatore)
136-137 Trichy Road
Coimbatore 641 045, T.N., India
Email: ayurveda@vsnl.com
Website: www.avpayurveda.com

Australian Institute of Ayurvedic Medicine
Dr. Frank Ros, Director
19 Bowey Avenue
Enfield S.A. 5085, Australia
Ph: 08-349-7303
Website: www.picknowl.com.au/homepages/suchi-karma

Australian School of Ayurveda
Dr. Krishna Kumar, MD, FIIM
27 Blight Street
Ridleyton, South Australia 5008
Ph. 08-346-0631

Ayur-Veda AB
Box 78, 285 22 Markaryd
Esplanaden 2, Sweden
Ph: 0433-104 90
Fax: 0433-104 92
Email: info@ayur-veda.se

Ayurveda Academy
Dr. P.H. Kulkarni, President
36 Kothrud, Opp. Mhatoba Temple
Pune 411 029, India
Ph: 91-212-332130
Fax: 91-212-363132/ 343933.
Email: ayurveda.academy@jwbbs.com

Ayurveda for Radiant Health & Beauty
Ivy Amar
16 Espira Court
Santa Fe, NM 87505
Ph: 505-466-7662
Website: www.ivyamar.com

Ayurvedic Holistic Center
Swami Sadashiva Tirtha, Director
82A Bayville Ave.
Bayville, NY 11709
Website: www.ayurvedahc.com

Ayurvedic Institute and Wellness Center
Dr. Vasant Lad, Director
11311 Menaul, NE
Albuquerque, NM 87112
Ph: 505-291-9698
Website: www.ayurveda.com

California Association of Ayurvedic Medicine
Website: www.ayurveda-caam.org

California College of Ayurveda
1117A East Main Street
Grass Valley, CA 95945
Ph: 530-274-9100
Email: info@ayurvedacollege.com
Website: www.ayurvedacollege.com
Two year state approved program in Ayurveda

The Chopra Center
David Simon
Deepak Chopra LLC
At La Costa Resort and Spa
2013 Costa Del Mar Road
Carlsbad, CA 92009-6801
Ph: 760-494-1600
Toll Free: 888-424-6772
Fax: 760-494-1608
Website: www.chopra.com

Diamond Way Ayurveda
PO Box 13753
San Luis Obispo, CA 93406
Ph: 805-543-9291
Website: www.diamondwayurveda.com

John Douillard
Life Spa, Rejuvenation through Ayurveda
3065 Center Green Dr.
Boulder, CO 80301
Ph: 303-442-1164
Website: www.LifeSpa.com

European Institute of Vedic Studies
Atreya Smith, Director
Editions Turiya
I.E.E.V sarl
B.P. 4
30170 Monoblet, France
Ph: (33) 466 85 04 11
Fax: (33) 466 85 0542
Website: www.atreya.com
Website: www.ayurvedicnutrition.com
Ayurvedic training in Europe

Ganesha Institute
Pratichi Mathur, President
4898 El Camino Real, Suite 203
Los Altos, CA 94022
Ph: 615-961-8316
Website: www.healingmission.com

Himalayan Institute
952 Bethany Turnpike, Building 2
Honesdale, PA 18431
Website: www.himalayaninstitute.org

Institute for Wholistic Education
Dept. NP
3425 Patzke Ln.
Racine, WI 53405
Ph: 262-619-1798
Website: www.wholisticinstitute.org

International Academy of Ayurveda
Dr. Avinash Lele
Nand Nandan, Atreya Rugnalaya
M.Y. Lele Chowk
Erandawana, Pune
411 004, India
Ph/Fax: 91-212-378532/524427
Email: avilele@hotmail.com
Website: www.ayurveda-int.org

International Yoga Studies
Sandra Kozak, Director
692 Andrew Court
Benicia, CA 94510
Ph: 707-745-5224
Email: IYSUSA@aol.com.
Website: internationalyogastudies.com

Kaya Kalpa International
Dr. Raam Panday
111 Woodster Rd.
Satto, NY 10012

Kayakalpa
Sri Tatwamasi Dixit
22/2 Judge Jumbulingam Road
Off Radhakrishnan Salai, Mylapore
Chennai 600 004, India
Website: www.mypandit.com

Dr. Avinash Lele
Atreya Rugnalaya
Erandwana, Pune
411 004, India
Tel/Fax: 91-20-5678532
Email: avilele@hotmail.com

Life Impressions Institute
Donald Van Howten, Director
613 Kathryn Street
Santa Fe, NM 87501
Ph: 505-988-2627

Light on Ayurveda: Journal of Health
Genevieve Ryder, Editor/Publisher
418-77 Quinaquisset Avenue
Mashpee, MA 02649
Ph: 508-477-4783
Website: www.loaj.com

Light Institute of Ayurveda
Dr.'s Bryan & Light Miller
PO Box 35284
Sarasota, FL 34242
Email: earthess@aol.com
Website: www.ayurvedichealings.com

Lotus Ayurvedic Center
4145 Clares St., Suite D
Capitola, CA 95010
Ph: 408-479-1667
Website: www.lotusayurveda.com

Lotus Press
Dept. NP
PO Box 325
Twin Lakes, WI 53181 USA
Ph: 262-889-8561
Fax: 262-889-2461
Email: lotuspress@lotuspress.com
Website: www.lotuspress.com
Publisher of books on Ayurveda, Reiki, aromatherapy, energetic healing, herbalism, alternative health and U.S. editions of Sri Aurobindo's writings.

Dr. Aldo Lubrano
Cursos de Medicina Ayurveda
Offers Dr. Frawley's trainings in Spanish
1452 Boston Post Road # 4K
Larchmont, New York, 10538
Ph: (914) 834 2836
Email: recepcion@lubrano.com
Website: www.lubrano.com

Midwest Institute of Vedic Studies
4230 N. Oakland Avenue, Suite 201
Shorewood WI 53211-2042
Website: Midwestinstituteofvedicstudies.com
Email:vedicinstitute@wi.rr.com

National Association of Ayurvedic Medicine
Website: www.ayurvedic-association.org

National Institute of Ayurvedic Medicine
584 Milltown Road
Brewster, NY 10509
Ph: 845-278-8700
Email: niam@niam.com
Website: www.niam.com

Dr. Subhash Ranade
Rajbharati, 367 Sahakar Nagar 1
Pune 411 009, India
Email: sbranade@hotmail.com

Rocky Mountain Institute of Yoga and Ayurveda
PO Box 1091
Boulder, CO 80306
Ph: 303-499-2910
Email: rmiya@earthnet.net
Website: www.rmiya.org

Sanskrit Sounds - Nicolai Bachman
PO Box 4352
Santa Fe, NM 87502
Email: shabda@earthlink.net
Website: www.SanskritSounds.com

Vinayak Ayurveda Center
2509 Virginia NE, Suite D
Albuquerque, NM 87110
Ph: 505-296-6522
Website: www.vinayakayurveda.com

Vedic Cultural Fellowship
Howard Beckman, Director
HC 70, Box 620
Pecos, NM 87552
Ph: 505-757-6194
Website: www.vedicworld.org

Wise Earth School of Ayurveda
Bri. Maya Tiwari
90 Davis Creek Road
Candler, NC 28715
Ph: 828-258-9999
Website: www.wisearth.org

Ayurvedic Herbal Suppliers

Auroma International
Dept. NP
PO Box 1008
Silver Lake, WI 53170 USA
Ph: 262-889-8569
Fax: 262-889-2461
Email: auroma@lotuspress.com
Website: www.auromaintl.com
Importer and master distributor of Auroshikha Incense, Chandrika
Ayurvedic Soap and Herbal Vedic Ayurvedic products.

Ayur Herbal Corporation
PO Box 6390
Santa Fe, NM 87502
Ph: 262-889-8569
Website: www.herbalvedic.com
Manufacturer of Herbal Vedic Ayurvedic products.

Ayush Herbs, Inc.
10025 N.E. 4th Street
Bellevue, WA 98004
Ph: 800-925-1371

Banyan Trading Company
PO Box 13002
Albuquerque, NM 87192
Ph: 505-244-1880; 800-953-6424
Website: www.banyantrading.com
Traditional Ayurvedic Herbs – Wholesale

Bazaar of India Imports
1810 University Avenue
Berkeley, CA 94703
Ph: 800-261-7662; 510-548-4110
Website: www.bazaarofindia.com

Bio Veda
215 North Route 303
Congers, NY 10920-1726
Ph: 800-292-6002

Earth Essentials Florida
Dr.'s Bryan and Light Miller
4067 Shell Road
Sarasota, FL 34242
Ph: 941-316-0920
Email: earthess@aol.com
Website: www.ayurvedichealings.com

Florida Vedic Institute/Universal Yoga
Baba Hari Nam Prem, Director
420 East S.R. 434 Suite D. Longwood FL 32750
E-mail: universalyoga@netzero.net
Website:www.floridavedicinstitute.com

Frontier Herbs
PO Box 229
Norway, IA 52318
Ph: 800-669-3275

HerbalVedic Products
PO Box 6390
Santa Fe, NM 87502
Website: www.herbalvedic.com

Internatural
Dept. NP
PO Box 489
Twin Lakes, WI 53181 USA
800-643-4221 (toll free order line)
262-889-8581 (office phone)
262-889-8591 (fax)
Email: internatural@lotuspress.com
Website: www.internatural.com
Online and mail retailer of Ancient Secrets Nasal Cleansing Pot,
Himalayan Institute Neti Pot, Sinu-Cleanse System and more.

Lotus Brands, Inc.
Dept. NP
PO Box 325
Twin Lakes, WI 53181 USA
Ph: 262-889-8561
Fax: 262-889-2461
Email: lotusbrands@lotuspress.com
Website: www.lotusbrands.com
Original supplier of the Ancient Secrets Nasal Cleansing Pot.

Lotus Herbs
1505 42nd Ave., Suite 19
Capitola, CA 95010
Ph: 408-479-1667
Website: www.lotusayurveda.com

Lotus Light Enterprises
Dept. NP
PO Box 1008
Silver Lake, WI 53170 USA
800-548-3824 (toll free order line)
262-889-8501 (office phone)
262-889-8591 (fax)
Email: lotuslight@lotuspress.com
Website: www.lotuslight.com
Wholesale distributor supplying stores and practitioners including Ancient Secrets Nasal Cleansing Pot, Himalayan Institute Neti Pot, Sinu-Cleanse System and more.

Maharishi Ayurveda Products International
417 Bolton Road
PO Box 541
Lancaster, MA 01523
Info: 800-843-8332 Ext. 903
Order: 800-255-8332 Ext. 903

Om Organics
3245 Prairie Avenue, Suite A
Boulder, CO 80301
Ph: 888-550-VEDA
Website: www.omorganics.com

Organic India
Affiliate of Om Organics
Indira Nager, Lucknow,
Uttar Pradesh, 226 016, India
Website: www.organicindia.com

Planetary Formulations
PO Box 533
Soquel, CA 95073
Website: www.planetherbs.com
Formulas by Dr. Michael Tierra

Tri Health
Jeff Lindner, director, Kauai, Hawaii
Ph: 800-455-0770
Email: oilbath@aloha.net
Website: www.oilbath.com
Ayurvedic herbs and formulas from the Kerala Ayurvedic Pharmacy

4.
Author's Information

Dr. David Frawley (Pandit Vamadeva Shastri) is a world recognized teacher of Vedic knowledge, working in the related fields of Yoga, Ayurvedic medicine and Vedic astrology for the past thirty years. He has written over thirty books on these topics and trained numerous students in their practice. He is currently the director of the American Institute of Vedic Studies in Santa Fe, New Mexico.

The American Institute of Vedic Studies

The Institute is an educational and research center, offering courses, publications and resources for those wanting a deeper knowledge of the Vedic tradition. The Institute conducts three important distant learning programs, a foundation course in Ayurvedic medicine, an advanced Yoga and Ayurveda course (recently introduced) and a foundation course in Vedic astrology. The Institute also offers advanced tutorial training and has affiliated organizations in the United States, Europe and India. Please contact our website for more information and for our newsletter.

American Institute of Vedic Studies
PO Box 8357, Santa Fe NM 87504-8357
Dr. David Frawley (Pandit Vamadeva Shastri), Director
Ph: 505-983-9385, Fax: 505-982-9156
Website: www.vedanet.com
Email: vedicinst@aol.com

5.
Endnotes

[1] While sounding similar, it is not the same term as neti meaning negation, as in neti, neti, 'not this, not that' of yogic philosophy.

[2] Note the *Yoga Sutras* of Patanjali for more information, particularly its second section or pada.

[3] This is not only to promote health and awareness, but to reduce the amount of violence in the world.

[4] Such as Yoga Upanishads like *Pingala, Yogashikha, Yogakundali, Paingala, Shandilya,* and *Jabaladarshana.*

[5] The Kundalini or serpent power of Yoga itself is a type of awakened Prana.

[6] The main source book of Hatha Yoga is the *Hatha Yoga Pradipika.*

[7] Note the author's book *Yoga and Ayurveda* for more information on this topic.

[8] For example, the author's own *Ayurvedic Healing* has a very extensive such constitutional questionnaire that is also repeated in his *Yoga for Your Type.*

[9] This is why Prana connects to the Great God Shiva, the lord of the Yogis, in yogic thought. Shiva represents the supreme Prana from which all life and consciousness arises. Shiva is also regarded as the original guru (Adinath) of the Hatha Yoga tradition in ancient texts like the *Hatha Yoga Pradipika.*

[10] Technically in finger units or digits, anguli in Sanskrit (note *Ayurveda and Marma Therapy,* Frawley, Ranade, Lele)

[11] Ayurveda and Yoga recognize the existence of five Pranas. The Prana in the head is the master Prana among the five. Of the other Pranas each has its separate name and function. Udana, the upward moving pranic air, governs speech and effort. Apana, the downward moving pranic air, governs elimination and reproduction. Vyana, the outward moving pranic air, governs circulation and the extension of the limbs. Samana, the balancing pranic air, governs the process of digestion.

[12] In Ayurvedic medicine, the wrong use or functioning of the senses is one of the main causes of all diseases.

[13] Note Resource section in the back of the book.

[14] However, the lining of the colon does not have many nerve endings like the nose, so the use of enemas or colonics consisting only of water may not be experienced as irritating, even when they may damage the lining of the large intestine.

[15] Note bibliography for books on Pranayama that discuss these techniques.

[16] Such yogic suspension of the breath is very different than merely holding the breath. It requires opening up to a higher Pranic force at a deeper level of the mind. I am not recommending anyone to simply try to hold their breath. Deep breathing must be developed first. Please consult a Yoga teacher who can help you with this process if you want to do it.

[17] Note Hatha Yoga Pradipika II.22-37.

[18] Or the Ayurvedic formula Trikatu (ginger, black pepper and long pepper).

[19] Pitta can also move downwards causing heat, inflammation and infection in the lower body.

[20] Jatamamsi has better tonifying and strengthening powers for the brain and nerves. Valerian is more of a sedative.

[21] Some Ayurvedic books refer to Bacopa as Brahmi and Hydrocotyle as Manduka parni. Generally the Bacopa is more tonifying and the Hydrocotyle is more cleansing in action.

[22] Note *Ayurveda and Marma Therapy* (Frawley, Ranade, Lele) for more information on these marma points and how to use them.

[23] As turmeric also functions as a yellow dye, be careful not to get it on your clothes!

[24] Like the author's *Ayurvedic Healing.*

[25] Vata caused polyps occur owing to dryness and irritation in the nose. They can be treated with oils like sesame and soothing and tonifying herbs. Pitta-caused nasal polyps result from heat and inflammation in the head and require a cooling therapy. Kapha caused polyps, which are the most common, occur from poor circulation and mucus accumulation. They can be treated by stimulating and detoxifying herbs and nasal therapies.

[26] What is called Ama in Ayurvedic thought.

[27] Ayurvedic herbs like Arjuna (Terminalia arjuna) and Guggul (Commiphora mukul).

[28] Many Ayurvedic herbs are helpful like Ashwagandha, Shatavari and Guduchi (Tinospora cordifolia).

6.
Index

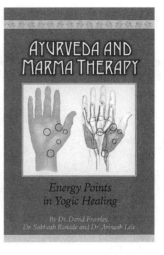

Ayurveda
Nature's Medicine
by Dr. David Frawley & Dr. Subhash Ranade

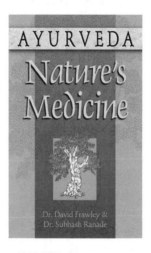

Ayurveda, Natures Medicine is an excellent introduction to the full field of Ayurvedic Medicine from diet and herbs to yoga and massage. It has a notable emphasis on practical self-care and daily life regimens that makes it helpful for everyone seeking health and wholeness. The book is an excellent primer for students beginning in the field and wanting to have a firm foundation to understand the entire system.

Trade Paper   ISBN 978-0-9149-5595-5   368 pp pb $19.95

Available at bookstores and natural food stores nationwide or order your copy directly by sending $19.95 plus $2.50 shipping/handling ($.75 s/h for each additional copy ordered at the same time) to:

Lotus Press, PO Box 325, Dept. AH, Twin Lakes, WI 53181 USA
toll free order line: 800 824 6396   office phone: 262 889 8561
office fax: 262 889 2461   email: lotuspress@lotuspress.com
web site: www.lotuspress.com

Lotus Press is the publisher of a wide range of books and software in the field of alternative health, including Ayurveda, Chinese medicine, herbology, aromatherapy, Reiki and energetic healing modalities. Request our free book catalog.

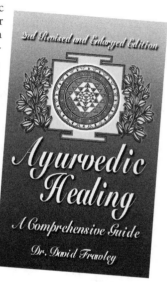

The Yoga of Herbs
An Ayurvedic Guide to Herbal Medicine
Second Revised and Enlarged Edition

by Dr. Vasant Lad & Dr. David Frawley

For the first time, here is a detailed explanation and classification of herbs, using the ancient system of Ayurveda. More than 270 herbs are listed, with 108 herbs explained in detail. Included are many of the most commonly used western herbs with a profound Ayurvedic perspective. Important Chinese and special Ayurvedic herbs are introduced. Beautiful diagrams and charts, as well as detailed glossaries, appendices and index are included.

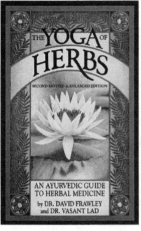

"Dr. Frawley and Dr. Lad have made a truly powerful contribution to alternative, natural health care by their creation of this important book. This book...will serve not only to make Ayurvedic medicine of greater practical value to Westerners but, in fact, ultimately advance the whole system of Western herbalism forward into greater effectiveness. I think anyone interested in herbs should closely study this book whether their interests lie in Western herbology, traditional Chinese herbology or in Ayurvedic medicine."

— Michael Tierra, Author, *The Way of Herbs*

Trade Paper   ISBN 978-0-9415-2424-7   288 pp   pb $15.95

Available at bookstores and natural food stores nationwide or order your copy directly by sending $15.95 plus $2.50 shipping/handling ($.75 s/h for each additional copy ordered at the same time) to:

Lotus Press, PO Box 325, Twin Lakes, WI 53181 USA
toll free order line: 800 824 6396   office phone: 262 889 8561
office fax: 262 889 2461   email: lotuspress@lotuspress.com
web site: www.lotuspress.com

Lotus Press is the publisher of a wide range of books and software in the field of alternative health, including Ayurveda, Chinese medicine, herbology, aromatherapy, Reiki and energetic healing modalities. Request our free book catalog.

Yoga & Ayurveda

Self-Healing and Self-Realization
by Dr. David Frawley

Yoga and Ayurveda together form a complete approach for optimal health, vitality and higher awareness. YOGA & AYURVEDA reveals to us the secret powers of the body, breath, senses, mind and chakras. More importantly, it unfolds transformational methods to work on them through diet, herbs, asana, pranayama and meditation. This is the first book published in the West on these two extraordinary subjects and their interface. It has the power to change the lives of those who read and apply it.

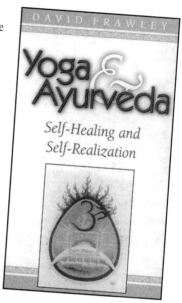

Dr. David Frawley (Vamadeva Shastri) is recognized both in India and the West for his knowledge of Vedic teachings, which include Ayurveda, Vedic Astrology, and Yoga. He is the author of twenty books published over the last twenty years, including Ayurveda and the Mind, Yoga of Herbs, Ayurvedic Healing and Astrology of the Seers. His Vedic translations and historical studies on ancient India have received much acclaim, as have his journalistic works on modern India.

Trade Paper   ISBN 978-0-9149-5581-8   360 pp $19.95

Available through your local bookseller or direct from:
Lotus Press, P O Box 325, Dept. NP, Twin Lakes, WI 53181 USA
262-889-8561 (office phone)   262-889-2461 (office fax)   800-824-6396 (toll free order line)
email: lotuspress@lotuspress.com   web site: www.lotuspress.com

To Order send $19.95 plus $2.50 shipping/handling ($.75 for each additional copy) to Lotus Press.

Lotus Press is the publisher of a wide range of books in the field of alternative health, including Ayurveda, Chinese medicine, herbology, reiki, aromatherapy, and energetic healing modalities. Request our free book catalog.

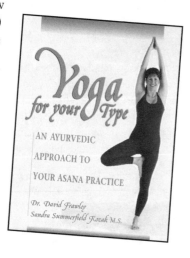